Women and Alcohol

Women and Alcohol

A Dangerous Pleasure

by Geraldine Youcha

Crown Publishers, Inc.
New York

Published by Crown Publishers, Inc., 225 Park Avenue South, New York, New York 10003

Originally published under the title *A Dangerous Pleasure* by Hawthorn Books, Inc.

CROWN is a trademark of Crown Publishers, Inc.

Manufactured in the United States of America

Library of Congress Cataloging-in-Publication Data

Youcha, Geraldine.
  Women and alcohol.

  Rev. ed. of: A dangerous pleasure. c1978.
  Bibliography: p.
  Includes index.
  1. Women—United States—Alcohol use.   I. Youcha,
Geraldine.   Dangerous pleasure.   II. Title.   III. Title:
Women and alcohol.   IV. Title: Dangerous pleasure.
HV5137.Y68   1986   362.2'92   85-26977
ISBN 0-517-55978-1

10 9 8 7 6 5 4 3 2 1

First Revised Edition

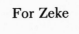

Contents

Preface

As a magazine writer and newspaper columnist, I see myself as a reporter of the social scene. Changing concerns about women and alcohol are certainly part of this picture. I am not a recovered alcoholic or the daughter of one, although many times in interviews for this book people have insisted that I must be.

My concern is for all women—those who don't drink at all, those who, like me, drink infrequently, and those who drink moderately or abusively. We share the same physiology and the same cultural commandments. What does alcohol do to us? And how do society's expectations and attitudes affect the way users and abusers are perceived and treated?

As a student during the 1940s at Northwestern University in Evanston, Illinois—the home of the Woman's Christian Temperance Union—I first became aware of the close interrelationship between women and this ubiquitous drug. I never attended any of the abstemious "catnip teas," since I was busy trying to learn to like beer, but exposure to the emotional coloring of attitudes about drinking was inescapable in that capital city of temperance.

This book is an attempt to provide information rather than polemics about a subject that triggers deeply personal responses. It brings together research, opinion, and human experience to present an up-to-date picture of what is known about how drinking affects women. As a reporter, not a scientist or therapist, I have tried to present the controversies as well as the few certainties.

For those who are interested in more details, there are footnotes and a bibliography at the end of the book. Since this is not meant to be a technical review of the literature, footnotes have been kept to a minimum. Most references can be found easily by matching the author's name, mentioned in the text, with the bibliography. Important studies not specifically identified have been footnoted. And, of course, there is a lot of previously unpublished material that was gathered in interviews, at scientific meetings, and at forums discussing the place of alcohol in women's lives.

It would be impossible to thank personally all the people across the country—researchers, educators, counselors, alcoholic women, recovering alcoholics, and social drinkers—who were generous with their time and knowledge. But there are a few who were especially helpful in reading part or all of the manuscript and offering their comments: Sheila Blume, Edith Gomberg, Susan Gordon, Ben Morgan Jones, Burroughs Mitchell, and Frank Seixas.

Women
and
Alcohol

1

Superior But Not Equal

The notion that woman is on a pedestal and falls farther than man when she drinks more than she can gracefully hold requires a ritualistic bow. Once this has been done, most writers hurry on without looking too closely at the base of the monument. If they poked around, they would find engraved on the column these time-encrusted injunctions, for women only: Be better than I am. Be the guardian of moral and social values. Be beautiful. Through the centuries these commandments, preserved by men's needs, have affected the way women are seen whenever they raise glasses of good cheer to their lips. And although times have changed, attitudes have altered very little.

"Thou shalt be better than I am" was summed up this way by the seventeenth-century dramatist Thomas Otway: "O Woman! lovely woman! Nature made thee To temper man; we had been beasts without you." Frances Willard, leader of the temperance crusade, also had no doubt that men needed women to show them the way. From her pinnacle of righteousness, she said woman was "above [man] on the hard-won heights of purity that she may lead him upward. . . ." Miss Willard was caught up in the Victorian age, which could afford to see its females as just a little lower than the angels, and certainly better than men.

As historian Gerda Lerner explains, "What was new in the

1830's was the cult of the lady, her elevation to a status symbol. The advancing prosperity of the early nineteenth century made it possible for middle-class women to aspire to the status formerly reserved for upper-class women. The 'cult of true womanhood' of the 1830's became a vehicle for such aspirations. Mass circulation newspapers and magazines made it possible to teach every woman how to elevate the status of her family by setting 'proper' standards of behavior, dress and literary tastes. *Godey's Lady's Book* and innumerable gift books and tracts of the period all preach the same gospel of 'true womanhood'—piety, purity and domesticity." Of course, outside the domestic sphere, she had no function. She was clearly morally superior and just as clearly politically and intellectually inferior. Unlike men, she never overindulged in anything—not alcohol, not sex. The latter was an inconvenience to be borne on the way to motherhood. And only a fallen woman drank more than a ritual glass of wine.

For men, sexual and drinking scoreboards have been a standard way of expressing masculinity. But, despite the current popularity of books and novels about women's sexual exploits and fantasies, the double standard is still there; a good woman doesn't hang her successes on her belt like scalps. When two women students at the Massachusetts Institute of Technology published a sexual rating sheet of their thirty-six ex-lovers, naming names, they were swiftly disciplined for overstepping the bounds of good taste and, of course, poaching on a male preserve. A decent woman doesn't drink enough to become too affectionate or sexually receptive, either. Although, as the experts insist, she won't do anything after a few drinks that she wouldn't do without them, alcohol makes it easier for her to act on her impulses.

Ogden Nash said it without the scientific jargon a long time ago:

> *Candy*
> *Is dandy*
> *But liquor*
> *Is quicker.* *

Some wag put it even more bluntly with a rewrite of another classic:

*"Reflections on Ice-Breaking,"copyright © 1930 by Ogden Nash. From *Verses from 1929 On* by Ogden Nash, by permission of Little, Brown and Company.

Men seldom make passes
At girls who wear glasses
So Dorothy Parker has writ.
But they pass at the lasses
Who empty their glasses.
Eh, Dorothy, isn't that it?*

The assumption that a woman who drinks—even a little—has questionable morals shows up very early in history. The Babylonians went to the trouble of pressing cuneiforms into a clay tablet with their own penalty for a woman who strayed: "If a priestess or a holy sister who has not remained in the convent shall open a wine shop or enter a wine shop for a drink, that woman shall be burned," the Code of Hammurabi grimly declared two thousand years before Christ. Some scholars insist that Babylonian wine shops were also brothels.

The ancient Greeks had drunken orgiastic rites—at first for women only—to honor Bacchus, the god of both wine and fertility. But these were strictly regulated religious celebrations, held only three times a year. They didn't alter attitudes toward women and drinking in ordinary, everyday life.

In ancient Rome a man could kill his wife if he smelled wine on her breath because "drinking inspires adultery." And it was hard for her to get away with even a sip. She was required to kiss all her male relatives, and all of her husband's, too, when they met for the first time on any day. She could hardly avoid testifying against herself if she had indulged in a forbidden drink. The aroma was enough. No other evidence was necessary.[1]

The elder Pliny, a historian of the first century after Christ, tells the horrifying tale of a married woman whose family kept her from eating until she starved to death because she had stolen the keys to the wine cellar.[2] Cruel and unusual punishment, perhaps, but the Romans and Hammurabi probably would have felt comfortable with the attitude of one small-city Southerner who recently told a newspaper reporter, "If a man goes into a bar and has a drink, no one blinks an eye. But let a woman do the same thing and she's automatically labeled a slut or worse." This venerable point of view can't be dismissed lightly as a regional aberration,

*Printed with permission of Melville Shavelson.

despite today's changing sexual and drinking mores. Like barna-
cles, old feelings encrust and complicate the way we look at behavior. In his review of the literature on alcoholic women,
psychiatrist Marc Schuckit observed of standards prevalent only a
few years ago, "Any woman seen alone in a bar was assumed to be
a prostitute, or at least a woman looking for a bed partner. By ex-
tension, any woman who was drunk, or even drinking, might have
been perceived in the same context." She was acting like a man,
not better than one. His vices could be assumed to be hers,
too.

Unlike some other nations, we have not only been reluctant to
allow women into public drinking places, we have also often denied them jobs there because they must be protected against men's
evil intentions and their own sexual susceptibility. In a 1948 opinion for the majority in which it was declared that a state could
prohibit women from acting as bartenders (*Goesart v. Cleary*), Supreme Court Justice Felix Frankfurter wrote, "The fact that
women may now have achieved virtues that men have long
claimed as their prerogatives and now indulge in vices that men
have long practiced, does not preclude the States from drawing a
sharp line between the sexes, certainly in such matters as the regulation of the liquor traffic. . . . The Constitution does not require
legislatures to reflect sociological insight or shifting social standards, any more than it requires them to keep abreast of the latest
scientific standards."

As a matter of fact, the latest scientific information might bolster the judicial (and ancient Roman) attitude about the sharp distinction between the sexes. To the dismay of feminists, recent
research on women's feelings after a few drinks indicates that alcohol does make a woman feel more feminine and sexy. And it
makes a man feel more powerful. The combination, as the ancients
observed, may lead to trouble. It's best to keep woman on her pedestal, out of reach and out of temptation. When she descends to
man's earthly level, she disturbs the equilibrium of society. "We
would rather have them in their place," sociologist Joseph Hirsh
observes, "which is another way of saying that they define and
make our own place possible and even more comfortable."[3]

There is more to woman's place than spiritual superiority. She is
also seen as the keeper of social and moral values, the one who
knows when to punish and when to hug. This is commandment

number two: Be the guardian of moral and social values. If she gets tipsy, a woman can hardly do her job as a mother, teacher of the young, and noble repository for all that is good. Researcher Joan Curlee puts it succinctly in her comparison of male and female alcoholic patients: "No one likes to believe that the hand that rocks the cradle might be a shaky one."

The expectation that woman will be the guardian of the young and the vehicle for passing on the moral laws of mankind goes back a long way. In the Midrash, an ancient commentary on the Old Testament, there is a story about God's hesitation in giving Moses the Ten Commandments. Before he revealed them, God insisted on having women present when they were to be shown to the people, because women were the ones who would pass his precepts on to future generations.[4] This time-honored responsibility for maintaining and conveying civilization's moral tone makes excessive drinking something to be condemned.

Drink also interferes with the third injunction: Be beautiful. This is a fairly recent requirement, going back only to the High Renaissance of the fifteenth century in Europe, but it has enormous force. In the Renaissance, instead of being treated as chattel or as a partner in producing the goods for the household, woman for the first time became a decorative object. She didn't have to work. She could spend her time putting potions on her skin to make it milk-white, dressing in jewel-encrusted velvet, and adorning the lord's manor house. When Emily Jane Putnam, first dean of Barnard College, examined the historical roles of women, she found that "the only positive demand made of the lady was that she be beautiful."

This injunction survived centuries, social changes, and economic upheavals. Although first directed at the upper-class woman, it filtered down (as most things do) to all layers of society. The beautiful woman became more than just an ornament—she became a status symbol for the man whose arm (and income) supported her. She spent hours (and money) preparing herself for this role, and when she failed, everyone close to her shared in her shame. Actress Jan Clayton, who was herself a recovering alcoholic, described society's reactions this way: "A drunk woman? A female lush? Intolerable. So let's be terribly quiet about it. And though the problem may not go away, perhaps she—a wife, a mother, a sweetheart, or even a daughter—will go, somewhere,

where there is no more embarrassment by this unattractive crea-
ture who is a dreadful reflection on all of us."

In the eyes of her family and friends, a woman who drinks too
much is not beautiful; she disobeys a clear commandment and is
fallen. Even a "nonjudgmental" alcoholism counselor described
one of her big-city neighbors as "disgusting" after she saw her try
to get out of a taxi following an afternoon of drinking. "She
sprawled in the doorway of the cab and her dress crept up to her
neck. She looked awful, and her poor husband kept trying to pick
her up." The woman, too, knows that she is not good to look at,
and this compounds her own feelings of self-loathing. Joy Baker, a
recovering alcoholic and the wife of former Senate majority leader
Howard Baker, remembers her own feelings about what happened
to her: "Your whole body is blah," she said. "It takes just one good
look in a full-length mirror, the puffy, balloon face, the bulbous
body that has no shape. Suddenly it hits you."

But the idealized woman (and the ideal is accepted by both
sexes) is good to look at, a virgin or at least a wife, the keeper of
social and moral values, and a totally virtuous mother. That's why
excessive drinking—or even drinking that might not be considered
excessive in a man—is both incredible and completely unaccept-
able.

As Frederick Lewis Allen explains in his classic study of the
twenties, *Only Yesterday:*

> Women were the guardians of morality; they were made of
> finer stuff than men and were expected to act accordingly.
> Young girls must look forward in innocence (tempered per-
> haps with a modicum of physiological instruction) to a roman-
> tic love match which would lead them to the altar and to
> living happily ever after. . . . And although the attitude toward
> smoking and drinking by girls differed widely in different
> strata of society and different parts of the country, majority
> opinion held that it was morally wrong for them to smoke and
> could hardly imagine them showing the effects of alcohol.

Attitudes about sex and smoking have changed more since then
than attitudes about intoxication. The male drunk is seen as funny:
Charlie Chaplin weaving down the street, or the cartoon comic
who mistakes a lamppost for a beautiful woman and whispers

sweet nothings to its unyielding center. The female drunk, on the other hand, is an embarrassment or, even worse, an object of pity and scorn. You're not expected to laugh at an inebriated woman. " 'Drunk as a lord,' " points out psychiatrist Sheila Blume, "is an expression of good cheer. Try saying 'Drunk as a lady.' "

The entertainment world has been aware of this difference for a long time. In Hollywood there used to be an actor who specialized in drunks. A director could call him up, he'd come in and play his three-minute scene, then leave. "You didn't have to explain why he was drinking or what happened to him later. He was just funny. You could never do that with a woman," longtime comedy writer and director Mel Shavelson explains. "For her, you'd have to pay for violating the rules."

Arthur Laurents, who wrote the 1977 hit movie *The Turning Point,* recognized this unwritten rule when he had his young ballet dancer play a brief, funny drunk scene during a performance. She had been drinking only because of the painful breakup of a love affair; in swift payment for her indulgence, she threw up.

What may be one of the few successful modern attempts to get prolonged laughs from a woman's excessive use of alcohol is Lucille Ball's hilarious drunk scene in Shavelson's movie *Yours, Mine and Ours.* She's come to meet the children of the man she loves; there are nine of them, and they're not interested in having a new mother. Surreptitiously they spike her ladylike one screwdriver before dinner, making it almost pure alcohol. By the time she sits down at the table she is off balance, giggly, and finally in tears. The strictures about drunkenness and unacceptability seem to evaporate in Miss Ball's zany portrayal as she dumps mashed potatoes into the lap of the child next to her, spills the milk, and makes futile attempts to clean up the mess. Shavelson says he had difficulty persuading her to play the scene, and her nervousness made the whole thing more realistic. But the laughs she got were not simple ones. The episode is acceptable—and funny—because it is accidental. The character didn't know what she was drinking. And the whole thing took place in private—family only—in the home, where women have often been permitted to drink in Western societies. The major taboos had been left untouched, and it was the dirty trick, not the drunkenness, that gave the audience permission to laugh. She didn't even suffer any consequences (beyond being sick, off camera, in the bathroom). The handsome suitor married her and the children learned to love her. One drunken episode doesn't make an alcoholic.

The portraits of women alcoholics—and there have been a few in movies—have sometimes shown them doing funny things, but there has usually been a sob beneath the antics. These women have often been shielded by those around them and whisked out of the way before they could make fools of themselves. The strictures against drunkenness in women, and the social stigma attached to it, have combined to protect the woman alcoholic from public view. As one Alcoholics Anonymous member, the wife of a prominent suburban doctor, explains, "I was protected almost until my death. No one wanted to notice what was happening to me." Dr. Ruth Oakley, unit director of the John Norris Clinic in Rochester, New York, went even further: "Men sometimes let their alcoholic wives die," she said, "rather than embarrass the family by bringing the problem into the open. It's the easy way out—and it happens."

Although the stigma is undoubtedly great for a woman, and it is obligatory in any discussion of alcoholism to emphasize it, Dr. Edith Gomberg of the University of Michigan School of Social Work reminds us that "society is down on all alcoholics, regardless of sex or previous condition of servitude." Although a man can boast about being stewed, he's not a figure to emulate if he is an alcoholic. A woman, though, loses her status as a role model much earlier, long before the end of the road.

The double standard—boys will be boys, but a woman who drinks too much has betrayed a sacred trust—has certainly caused a mountain of misery. Is there anything good to be said for it? Experts agree that there is one positive aspect to society's longstanding condemnation of excessive drinking in woman: Social pressure to stay away from alcohol saved some women from becoming addicted. But today women are rebelling against the constricting picture of themselves as goddesses entrusted with the morals of mankind. This may mean that alcoholism in women will increase. Or it may mean only that women with problems will feel less restrained about exposing themselves in public and trying to get help.

2

Drinking Habits

S ince World War II, women have been joining the drinking force at a faster rate than men. We are drinking earlier and more openly, rushing to erase the traditional differences. Probably the last time men's, women's, and children's drinking patterns were so nearly alike was in colonial days. Rum, then, was not a demon but a necessary part of daily living, like bread and cheese. Families downed the grog together as they now swallow vitamins. If they could afford it, they dosed themselves several times a day. Of course, men drank more—but women's drinking was not frowned on, and children were included too. Beer was so vital for survival that the Pilgrims settled at Plymouth instead of scouting for a more favorable spot, "for we could not take much time for further search and consideration, our victuals being much spent, especially beer."

In the nineteenth century, brewing and breadmaking moved out of the kitchen—women's sphere—into the factory, signaling a change in economics and in attitudes. Middle-class women, cut off from the production of alcohol, became temperance advocates. Men now went out to work and to drink; many of them could afford to support wives who, in other days, had shared in the economic chores and in the production and use of alcohol.

During Prohibition, in the 1920s, there was a trend back to

home consumption and home brewing—but World War I had sent women into the factories and offices and given them a taste of the world beyond their domestic domain. Prohibition introduced them to speakeasies and bathtub gin, and they never retreated to their old abstemious ways. "There has been a breakdown in the middle classes," a member of the Woman's Christian Temperance Union lamented after Repeal. "The upper classes have always used liquor. The lower classes have always used liquor. Now the middle class has taken over. The thing is slopping over from both sides."

World War II accelerated the change. From then until the mid-1970s, the percentage of women who drank at least once a month had risen from 45 percent to 66 percent (the rise was a slower 75 percent to 77 percent among men), and a 1977 Gallup poll showed that, although the proportion of men drinking stayed the same, the proportion of women rose 8 percent. Social equality is coming to mean equality of social drinking.

It's no wonder the percentage of women who drink is approaching that of men. We are becoming a unisex society—in clothes, in hair styles, in the way we spend our leisure time. As roles converge, so do drinking habits. But that isn't the whole story. Americans have been using recreational drugs more openly since the sixties, with only slight differences between young men and young women. Alcohol, scorned by this group at first, has gradually gained respectability. It has become the recreational drug of choice. In a national survey of teen-agers' attitudes by J. V. Rachal and his associates, only 28 percent of the young people agreed that "it is worse for a girl to drink than it is for a boy." The media, too, have contributed to the popularity of drugs. Television has taught us to pop something into our mouths to cure everything from the "the blahs" to "tired blood"; alcohol, if you believe the commercials, cures the greatest curse of all—loneliness. An attractive man is always in the picture.

We have also moved from the farms to the cities at an accelerating rate, and urban women have always been more likely to drink than their less sophisticated country cousins. And we are becoming more educated. As our college population has gone up, so has the proportion of women who drink. On-campus, publicly sanctioned (and often publicly supported) pubs and snack bars selling beer and wine were typical of colleges across the country in the 1970s, except for those in "dry" areas. Their acceptance reflected legal changes and a less straitlaced attitude about women drinking. In the 1980s, with the legal drinking age raised in many states, campuses started to "sober up," and many on-campus pubs closed. But women now commonly go into bars alone or in groups; singles bars welcome women as necessary to their existence (and sometimes offer half-price drinks as a come-on), and drinking has become the norm rather than the exception for a large, educated, urban population. Despite this narrowing of the gap, the double standard hasn't disappeared entirely; a woman will limit her drinking so she can drive home and allow her husband (or date) to drink as much as he likes. It's still unthinkable that the man would limit his intake so she can indulge herself. And, although the relaxation of the raised eyebrow when it comes to a woman with a glass in her hand has its advantages, it may also carry with it certain problems. Since drinking is no longer seen as deviant behavior for a woman, she is less protected than she used to be from social pressures to drink. Given similar pressures, she may develop similar drinking styles that push her toward equalizing the rates of problem as well as of social drinking. Studies have shown that a rise in the number of drinkers is accompanied by a rise in the number who drink excessively.

The phenomenon of men and women drinking together to any great extent is fairly new. W H. Pfautz's analysis of novels written between 1900 and 1904 showed men drinking alone or with other men in almost all the drinking scenes. Men and women were drinking together only 12 percent of the time in the Victorian age; by the mid-twenties, the percentage of mixed-sex drinking situations had soared to 40. As for women drinking with other women, it was a barely perceptible 0.4 percent of the time in the early novels, but had tripled by the middle of this century.

In the 1800s, women left the dining room to the men when brandy and cigars were passed around—partly to protect women from being exposed to drunken behavior and asphyxiation and, I suspect, at least as much to give the men time out from the strictures of Victorian propriety. As early as 1910, though, an upper-class clubwoman noted, "It has become a well-established habit for women to drink cocktails. It is thought the smart thing to do."

Mrs. Beeton, in her classic Edwardian compendium of household hints, *Beeton's Book of Household Management,* includes recipes for a martini and a Manhattan—sweeter than today's version in deference to untutored tastes. But most drinking was still a "males only" privilege.

American men were slower than their European counterparts to accept women as drinking partners. On the frontier, only women of a certain class (and you know what that was) were permitted in saloons and usually only through a side entrance marked "Family." Across the Atlantic, men and women drinking together was common long before the emancipation of women became an issue; in the United States, women marched for the vote at the turn of the century but were still largely abstainers socially.

It was, ironically, not until Prohibition that men were willing to let women join the party. But even so, some of the all-male drinking preserves didn't fall until antidiscrimination laws challenged their "men only" tradition half a century later.

The Men's Bar of the Biltmore Hotel in New York City was a grim holdout, where patrons would discourage women who wandered in by staring at them and then applauding until they walked out. In 1973 feminists challenged the men-only policy, and women were admitted. The place was never the same. One steady customer complained, "The men were so busy looking at the women, they didn't drink." The bar and the hotel have since closed.

The saga of the Biltmore illustrates the change in women's opportunities to drink openly. Well into the 1920s, many states made it illegal for women to stand at a bar, and some states prohibited women in bars (even at tables) unless accompanied by a male escort. As late as 1967, Amy Vanderbilt, arbiter of correct behavior, warned, "in the United States, unescorted women in bars, if indeed they are admitted, can expect trouble, and a lone woman drinker in a bar is frankly suspect." Now, of course, some of the barriers have fallen, making it easier for women to drink on their own schedule rather than on a man's. But a woman alone is still fair game, and the cocktail hour tradition is still strong; "I never drink until four o'clock in the afternoon," one career woman declared virtuously. One is tempted to rewrite Henry Wadsworth Longfellow's classic about the time spent with children to pinpoint the contemporary unwritten law:

Between the dark and the daylight
When the night is beginning to lower
Comes a pause in the day's occupations
That is known as the cocktail hour.

Why do people drink? There is compelling evidence that men drink to feel more manly and powerful, and that women drink to feel more feminine. Dr. Sharon Wilsnack, associate professor at the University of North Dakota Medical School, first looked into women's fantasies while a Harvard psychologist. She is now beginning to question whether the feminine "helplessness" some of her subjects then reported was really that or a reflection of the traditional way for women to get what they want—in other words, a female power strategy.

Masculinity and femininity aside, there are basic truths about mind-altering substances (and alcohol is probably the oldest): One sociologist summed them up with, "It keeps those happy who are already happy and makes the sad happy again." He might have added that these happy effects last for a short time. Alcohol is, as we shall see, a central nervous system depressant. Alfred Kazin, the literary critic, thinks that "like so many of the things we do to ourselves in this pill-happy culture, drinking is a form of technology. People drink for hereditary reasons, nutritional reasons, social reasons. They drink because they are bored, or tired or restless. People drink for as many reasons as they have for wanting to 'feel better.' " And the reasons people drink, psychologist John Jung found, affect how much they drink. Someone who drinks to escape from daily problems—to be "out of it"—is likely to drink more than one who drinks to celebrate—to be "with it."

The social command to drink, to have fun and be part of the gang, is a venerable one. An ancient tomb painting in Egypt shows servants urging women to "Drink to drunkenness. Drink! Do not spoil the entertainment."[1] In our own time, the award-winning actress Mercedes McCambridge sees this group pressure to drink this way: "People drink because being together makes them uncomfortable. What is the first thing anybody says to you when you go to a party? 'Hold on, sweetie, what will you have to drink?' Not 'Did your mother ever get over that terrible kidney trouble? Did you pay the rent? . . .' What will you have to drink, *because if you don't drink, what are we going to do with you all evening?"* Alcohol is a legendary social lubricant.

In psychological terms, what happens when people drink is what Dr. Edith Gomberg, a national authority on women and alcohol, calls a form of regressive behavior. We are able to be a little freer in speech, less cautious, more friendly or, at other times, less friendly; in other words, we can behave a little more as we did when we were children, before the process of socialization taught us to control and to mask feelings to a greater or lesser extent. It is an adaptive sort of regressive behavior because such a return to more childlike behavior is more or less acceptable under social drinking conditions in our society. Apparently many people need and seek such releases occasionally.

Americans have devised a unique vehicle for this accepted "time out" from adult behavior: the cocktail party. Dr. Morris Chafetz, the first head of the National Institute on Alcohol Abuse and Alcoholism, sees this standing up and drinking ritual as unhealthy. "It is a contribution to the world's drinking practices that I wish we had not made," he says flatly. In Europe, alcohol is an accompaniment to something else—usually a meal. In America, alcohol is the reason for getting together. "Basically," one historian concluded, "Mediterranean Man considers wine as an integral part of his meal and a pleasant, but minor, adjunct to his conversation. Basically again, Gothic Man, when he thinks of wine, considers a carouse." Americans owe a lot to the Goths. Dr. Ben Morgan Jones, a research psychologist who studies social drinkers, says, "The cocktail party may rank as the commonest form of organized drug-taking in the Western world."

We say "Come over for a drink" and everyone understands that the drink is not coffee or tea. This emphasis on drinking as a thing in itself goes back a long way. On the frontier, it was a man's prerogative, and although he drank in a barroom with others, each prototypical Gary Cooper was essentially alone, a rugged individualist. The American virtues of speed (swallow as many as you can as fast as you can) and competitiveness (my hollow leg is bigger than your hollow leg) were enshrined in myth and reality. In contrast, the fact that drinking on the European continent usually took place in a setting with women and children tended to keep it moderate and toned down what an observer of American habits called "the grim determination to have a good time 'even if it kills you.' "

Some of these attitudes have filtered from men to women, but women, even alcoholics, still drink less than their male counterparts, and drink differently. Patterns also vary with age, socioeconomic group, religion, and environment.

Some groups have firmly resisted the increasing pressures to "take a cup of kindness." These tend to be rural or small-town, old-stock Protestants. Their contrary traditions die hard, as hard as the ones we inherited from the frontier.

Former President Jimmy Carter, who certainly moved in social strata far from his abstemious Plains, Georgia, beginnings, ran a White House without hard liquor. "It's really kind of funny to me to see people kind of squirm because we don't serve liquor in the White House," Rosalynn Carter told a newspaper reporter. "I don't object to anybody drinking. They can drink if they want to, but if I don't want to serve liquor in the White House I don't have to do it, and I don't want to."

In some parts of the South, and in strictly Mormon Utah, abstention is the rule. One Plains, Georgia, resident, however, indicates that the rule is often bent. "Most everybody 'round here drinks," Collins Sullivan, a straight-talking lumber dealer says, "some more than others, of course, and most everybody 'round here goes to church, some more than others, of course, and all the churches say it's something you ought not to do, so most everybody who does pretends they don't."

But the churches may find soon that it's time to change their attitudes. An early warning signal came when teetotaler and fundamentalist preacher Billy Graham announced, "I do not believe that the Bible teaches teetotalism. Jesus drank wine. Jesus turned water into wine at a wedding feast. That wasn't grape juice as some of them try to claim."

Although Bible Belt women are more likely to be abstainers than others (in general, weekly church-going Protestant women are likely to be teetotalers or infrequent drinkers), the South didn't have a representative on the government listing of "soberest states." Basing their ratings on demographics such as age, urban-rural population, sex, religion, and income the National Institute on Alcohol Abuse and Alcoholism came up with a listing to provide the basis for allocating treatment funds. In the 1970s, *Fortune* magazine[2] irreverently characterized the plan as "states with more drunks get more money." According to this rating, the five drunkest areas, in descending order, were Alaska, the District of Columbia, Hawaii, California, and Washington. The soberest (generally more rural) were Iowa, Minnesota, Nebraska, South Dakota, and North Dakota. It's safe to assume that women follow men's leads in these states, and that Alaska's compulsive female drinkers would hardly feel comfortable in abstemious Iowa.

Cities and suburbs have more drinkers and more heavy drinkers than farms and small towns. San Francisco, called "Sodom and Gomorrah West" by columnist Herb Caen, won the tippling prize of the 1970s with 80 percent of its adult residents drinking; a startling 21 percent of the women ranked as heavy drinkers compared to 7 percent in other American cities, according to researcher Robin Room. By 1983, however, Washington, D.C., had moved into the top position, with an average alcohol consumption rate of 5.22 gallons a year as compared to the national average of 2.69. As a nation, though, we are a moderate twentieth on a list, compiled by the World Health Organization, of countries with the highest per capita consumption of alcohol. Luxembourg and then France head the list.

We are also more heterogeneous than most other countries, carrying with us customs and attitudes from other cultures that influence the way large groups of Americans use and abuse alcohol. Cultures using alcohol (particularly wine and beer) with food or in connection with family religious observances have fewer problems with drinking than those which separate it from mealtimes and see drinking as an excuse to get drunk. The French are a notable exception; although they drink wine with meals, they also have a dismally high rate of alcoholism. Lebanese, Italians, Chinese, Greeks, Spaniards, and Orthodox Jews, on the other hand, have low rates although they all consume respectable quantities of alcoholic beverages. These cultures have generally accepted ground rules about how much, where, and when alcohol may be used. Drunkenness is not funny; it is sad and somehow shameful. Children see their parents drink moderately and associate drinking with family occasions, rather than as an excuse for a wild time.

As usual, women follow in the footsteps of the men in these cultures—a few paces behind. In our own society, men are three to four times more likely to be heavy drinkers than women are, and anthropologist Donald Horton found this contrast even more evident in primitive societies. "Men are permitted to drink as much as they choose, but women are severely restricted as to the amount they may drink. In a few instances, women are prohibited entirely from drinking the alcoholic beverage even though they may be the ones who make it in the course of their preparation of food."

That women all over the world drink less than men may be due to more than cultural restrictions. The same thing happens in the animal kingdom. In some strains, male hamsters and rats drink more. And a study of man's close cousin, the chimpanzee, showed that, given free access to alcohol, twice as many males as females drank until they were drunk.[3]

When it comes to women's drinking patterns in this country, any attempt to tie them to ethnic groups has to be considered very carefully. As usual, only men have been studied, but there are other, more general, complications. For one thing, the melting pot has been at work for generations, making us as much a country of mongrels as of purebreds. For another, as men and women who trace their ancestry to one or another country in Europe, Asia, or Central or South America move into the mainstream of American life they adopt the attitudes of the majority about alcohol. This is a drinking culture; the abstainer is an oddity.

With these warnings in mind, it is still possible to get some idea of how different groups handle alcohol. Rosemary Aiello's family immigrated to this country from Sicily. Her mother was born here, yet repeated the patterns of the old country. Now in her sixties, she has drunk wine at dinner every day since she was nine years old. On weekends, if there are guests, and in deference to modern tastes, she may take a whiskey sour before dinner.

Rosemary drinks wine with dinner perhaps three times a week. The daily ritual has ended for her, but she drinks more cocktails than her mother (two or three times a week) even if there isn't company. This, of course, makes her more "American." She also has an occasional brandy nightcap. "Now that," she says, "is something my mother can't understand. Drinking has to go with eating."

Rosemary's daughters, the third generation born here, don't drink cocktails or beer (which their mother sometimes does to keep her husband company). Like their grandmother and great-grandmother, they stick to wine, occasionally with dinner, more often at wine-and-cheese parties. Unwittingly, as they reflect the modern trend toward moderation and the upsurge in the acceptance of wine by young people, they have returned to a variation of an old ethnic pattern. The power of the past, which provides attitudes as a base for action, has kept the family from problem drinking. But the picture is changing. Rosemary's experience fits the statistical finding that second- and third-generation Italians tend to drink more than those in Italy, adding beer and liquor (as she did) to the traditional wine. There is now early evidence (in a study by Dr. Howard T. Blane of Harvard) that men of Italian descent who have combined both culture patterns are having problems with alcohol.

Dr. Edith Gomberg points out that as people move out of close-knit immigrant communities into American life-styles, they adopt the customs of the people with whom they socialize. Social class, rather than ethnic background, then determines what the patterns will be.

The Jewish experience seems to bear this out. Jewish women are more likely to drink and less likely to be abstainers than other American women. (In an unlikely coupling, Jews share this distinction with Episcopalians.) For years, Orthodox Jews have been singled out as the group with the lowest percentage of problem drinkers in America. Now, as more and more of them move into secular lives, the protection offered by wine as part of daily religious ritual seems to be losing its force. There's no way to prove it, but the general impression is that Jews, too, are drinking more. And Dr. Sheila Blume, who has collected information about Jewish alcoholics for a research study, says that of the first seventy she talked to, a startling 50 percent were women.

Rabbi Issac Trainin of New York says that "hotels and caterers now report that Jews are drinking as much as non-Jews, and there are now more than twenty AA [Alcoholics Anonymous] groups in New York City that meet in temples, synagogues, and other Jewish institutions."

Certainly there is a trend toward "Americanization"—drinking what "real" Americans drink. For Jewish women, the movement into the larger culture pattern seems particularly hazardous. "There is a double identity crisis," says Esther, a member of AA. "If you're Jewish you can't drink too much; if you're a woman, you can't drink too much. If you drink too much you aren't Jewish and you aren't womanly. So what are you?"

Even though Jews are moving closer to other groups in their alcohol problem rates, no one is suggesting that, as one sociologist put it, "they are debauching themselves with drink." Rather, attitudes are changing, but it takes a long time for changes to become effective. Oriental-American women, another slow-to-assimilate group, are still less likely to drink as much as their white counterparts, even if both have college educations. (Part of this difference may be accounted for by a physiological, rather than a cultural factor. As Dr. Peter Wolff has shown, many Orientals have unpleasant reactions to small doses of alcohol, including flushing and heart palpitations.) But certainly cultural attitudes reinforce this genetic protection. In Japan, women consume only 10 percent of the country's alcohol and have traditionally been nondrinkers. But even Japan is beginning to change. Westernized Maki Hrashima, a Tokyo office worker in her twenties, visits a bar once a week, usually alone. "My older brother told me that I shouldn't come to such places," she told an interviewer, "but I like the mood here. Besides I haven't run into any weirdos."

Why the Irish, in particular, should be so prone to drinking problems has engaged the interest of many experts. They have concluded that the Irish (at home and in America) run into trouble for three basic reasons: Drinking (and the drink is whiskey) is part of every important rite of passage, from birth to marriage to death. Second, it is separated from eating and religion (although wine is used in celebrating the mass, it is usually only the priest who drinks) and third, the utilitarian value attached to whiskey can hardly be overestimated. Whiskey is a cure for homesickness, fevers, hunger, the ague, toothache, a hangover, and the exhaustion that follows hard labor. Going in search of a drink is a perfect excuse for escaping the nagging of women. Everybody does it; there is no anxiety attached to it. As usual, women are affected by these attitudes, accepting the role of whiskey as a medical and social necessity and drinking it themselves. Unfortunately, there are no studies of Irish-American women; they, like most other women, have been invisible to researchers.

As for American Indian women, Wanda Frogg, a Cree, who directed the North American Indian Women's Council on Chemical Dependency, estimated that an appalling 60 percent of Native

American women are alcoholic. But there are conflicting impressions. Some observers of life on and off the reservation reinforce the old stereotype of the Indian as particularly prone to alcohol problems. (They are usually talking about men.) Others report less drinking by Indians than by other segregated, economically deprived groups, although cirrhosis of the liver—the paradigmatic alcoholic disease—is eight times more prevalent among Indians than in the general population.[4] That Indians are particularly sensitive to the effects of alcohol is also being questioned. An article by L. J. Benion and T. K. Li in the respected *New England Journal of Medicine* reports they are no more susceptible genetically than any other group. About black women, too, there is very little information, although there is a hint that they may equal black men in rates of alcoholism.[5]

In contrast to the scarcity of data about minority and poor women (except for those in prisons and hospitals), there is a fair amount of information about the drinking habits of mostly middle-class white housewives and career women. Most of the information comes from knock-on-the-door surveys by publishers and pollsters trying to convince advertisers that women really do drink, or by social scientists examining the occasions and places in which drinking occurs. The results have to be looked at with a skeptical eye. As the Newspaper Advertising Bureau commented after conducting a three-city survey on wine, beer, and liquor usage and habits, "It has been found that many people are reluctant to discuss their personal drinking habits with interviewers." It seems easier to get frank answers about sex than about drinking. Marty Mann, founder of the National Council on Alcoholism, put it even more directly: "You can't take a census on drinking. If the census taker rang the bell and asked questions there'd be black eyes instead of answers."

Nevertheless, researchers keep trying. One is the social psychologist Thomas Harford, who is convinced that his survey in Boston in the summer of 1974 at least suggests what women's drinking patterns really are. Dr. Harford and his colleagues looked at what they call "contextual patterns." When do women drink? Where? With whom? Their theory is that drinking is "situationally specific" rather than individually determined. Obviously, if you go to a party you are more likely to drink than if you go to a movie. And, even though the past ten years have seen women's drinking patterns moving closer and closer to men's, the differences that exist are based largely on cultural attitudes plus the limited number of drinking situations to which women are still exposed.

He found, for example, that women are more likely to do most of their drinking on weekends—a time for parties, weddings, and other celebrations. They don't down quick ones at the bar; they drink when the occasion lasts more than an hour, and they're more likely to drink in a home (theirs or a friend's) or in a restaurant. Women drink more frequently at mealtimes, when their husband or another man is around. Men, on the other hand, spread their drinking around. They drink while playing ball, during a lunch-break at work, watching television, and at other times during the week.

Actually, differing life-styles provide the context for different drinking habits. There is a whole group of suburban women who gear their drinking to the train schedules, even though they're not the commuters. Every night, they fix drinks to be ready for their husbands and wait to unwind together. Sometimes, though, they run into trouble. If the train is late, their drinking accelerates— they may have a drink before the husband gets home, then another when he arrives, and dinner may never be served. Women who work in a field where business lunches are the rule, and a drink is part of lunch, may find that they are drinking more than they used to. One executive in an accounting firm—a man's world—finds she has to watch herself now that she's higher on the success ladder. "I drink at lunch if I'm with somebody else, but I don't drink at all if I'm by myself. And I may or may not have a drink or two when I get home. I try to give myself some dry times, because I got scared when I'd wake up in the morning and ask my husband, 'Who did the dishes last night?' Of course I'd remember when he said, 'You did,' but that was enough to make me careful."

Michael Korda, author of *Success! How Every Man and Woman Can Achieve It*, sees alcohol as a lot less important than it used to be in the business world, partly because women are in positions of power. There are still after-work drink dates but "the martini . . . has long since been replaced by the glass of white wine, the spritzer (wine and soda) and Perrier water with a slice of lime. It's not so much that people have turned away from alcohol for any moralistic reasons; it's simply that most people are trying to lose weight and know that nothing puts it on like three stiff drinks."

Time magazine has dubbed the trend away from hard liquor and hard drinking, "the new temperance."

Working women in clerical jobs or the traditional "pink collar" occupations may find that working makes no difference in where or how much they drink. Like women at home, their drinking is confined mostly to weekends. Some high-pressured working women, however, adopt the traditional masculine pattern. "I unwind with two martinis every night before dinner," a college professor says. "And I'm not an alcoholic," she adds quickly.

This variation in acceptable patterns is what makes it hard to define moderate drinking. Psychiatrist Sheila Blume, an expert on women and problem drinking, says, "First tell me a woman's socioeconomic class, whether she spends her days at home with the kids, in a career or a job, how much her husband and friends drink. Of course," she adds impishly, "the standard definition of moderate drinking is 'what I drink, or maybe a little less.' "

For his massive study of American drinking practices, sociologist Don Cahalan developed a complex scale using both quantity and frequency in his calculations. According to his standards, someone can be a moderate drinker and drink two drinks a day, but never more than two drinks on any one occasion. A heavy drinker, on the other hand, drinks every day or almost every day and, on occasion, has five or more drinks. Women who drink are overwhelmingly light or infrequent drinkers; many of them drink once a month or less, and more than 30 percent of American women don't drink at all.

All this, like most sociology, is dedicated to documenting the obvious. But the documentation is valuable because it provides a way to correct myths that have become widespread and distort the true picture of women's drinking habits. Dr. Harford found, for example, that contrary to conventional wisdom, women aren't more likely to drink alone. Men are. He is quick to point out that he is talking about social drinking, not alcoholism. "Probably the woman who has a problem starts to hide it," he says. "She ends up drinking alone. She doesn't start that way." Dr. Eileen Corrigan, a researcher at Rutgers University School of Social Work, says her studies support this. "Women do a lot of drinking alone after they are drinking very heavily. They may still drive everybody home from the party, then drink themselves into a stupor in their own living room. Women at home change their whole pattern of living to accommodate to their drinking, and if they're drinking a lot they tend to cut themselves off from other people and that intensifies the isolation."

Don Mills, an Ontario, Canada, entrepreneur probably knows more about the secret drinking of isolated women than many professionals in the field. He runs Dial-a-Bottle. All a woman has to do is phone in her order and, for a two-dollar fee, he picks it up from a licensed store and delivers it to her doorstep—legally. A lot of his customers, he says, are "little old ladies who don't want their neighbors to see them headed for the liquor store."

Statistically, divorced, single, and separated (but not widowed) women are more likely to drink heavily and alone. Also likely to drink heavily are members of a newly recognized group—women who are "cohabiting" without being married. The two peaks for all women drinking, according to Dr. Cahalan, are ages twenty-one to twenty-four, the working and dating period, and forty-five to forty-nine, the lonely time. The younger single woman is not worried about taking care of small children; she can drink without neglecting her responsibilities. At the later age level, the increase in drinking is often pinned on "the empty nest" and other stresses of middle age. Women without a man in the house are likely to drink alone; not necessarily for any deep psychological reason, but simply because there is no one else around.

And yet there may be more to it than that. One forty-ish divorced woman with a glamour job in television and two children sees the psychological pressures of single life hovering behind her increased consumption. She says ruefully, "I know someone who says Women's Lib all started when men decided they didn't want to live with the same woman for fifty years. Now there are a lot of women alone, and we have to make it work. Divorced women is where the action is. Hard drinking starts when you're left alone with the kids and all the responsibilities and no none to talk to."

Dr. Harford also noticed what other researchers have documented, that drinking—quantity, frequency, and occasion—changes with age. This means that for every individual, drinking has a natural history; a beginning, a middle, and often an end. Young women are more likely to drink than older women, but problems caused by drinking seem to be concentrated among women in their thirties and forties. After about age fifty, the amount a woman drinks goes down and the number of abstainers goes up. This is true in other cultures, too. Sociologist R. Sadour, looking at French drinking habits, grumbled, "Among women, preferences for all forms of alcohol—even champagne—decreased steadily with age." Interesting enough, in Boston, at least, the number of drinking occasions increases with increasing age. These are less likely to be parties or family celebrations, more likely to be drinks at home, at mealtime, with relatives. As the social world shrinks, celebrations fade into the past and so does "social" drinking. The quantity consumed at one time becomes small, the frequency high.

Economics and health, too, play a part. Limited incomes mean limited alcohol. One widow explained, "If I'm going to drink at all it has to be the best, and I just don't have the money any more to buy good Scotch." If cost doesn't do it, doctor's orders often put a stop to the use of alcohol, since increasing age may mean diabetes, heart disease, or other chronic conditions that don't mix well with liquor.

Whatever their age, women college graduates are most likely to drink, and the trend of other groups to adopt the patterns of the top of the heap may mean, inevitably, that more and more women will be using alcoholic beverages. Women who started college and never finished are more likely to be heavy drinkers than any other group—including those with a high school education or less. Dr. Cahalan also found in his national study of drinking practices that there are more abstainers among lower-class women—those in service and factory jobs, close to the bottom of the educational and economic scale—but also a significant proportion of heavy drinkers. A working-class woman who drinks at all is likely to drink a lot.

This part of the equation fits the stereotype of the poor, hard-drinking woman—but the number of abstainers comes as a surprise. Contrary to popular myth, the proportion of heavy drinkers goes up from 6 percent of people with an eighth-grade education to 15 percent of college graduates. Evidently people with lower-paying jobs, and less money to spend for fun, spend less on liquor.

Despite the fact that there are more heavy drinkers among the upper classes, the drunken lower-class woman continues to be a standard feature of folklore and fiction. Eliza Doolittle, *My Fair Lady*'s cockney heroine, reported that her aunt was revived from certain death with a spoonful of gin. When an elegant Englishwoman was shocked by this remedy, Eliza replied indignantly, "Gin was mother's milk to her."

In 1902 Henry James noticed that "drink stands to the poor and unlettered in the place of symphony concerts and literature." At that time in England, women were reported to be drinking more than before and fistfights and hatpin (a potent weapon) bouts erupted on the streets. In the cities, the average working-class family spent six shillings a week on alcohol—"a terrifying figure," according to the historian Marghanita Laski.[6]

In this country, too, there is a tradition linking working-class women and heavy drinking. Particularly among some immigrant groups there were few evening pleasures, and women were as welcome as men in the neighborhood taverns. As Patricia Sexton, brought up in a blue-collar community, recalled in a *Harper's* magazine article, "My mother has never palled around with the girls or been any part of the coffee klatch circuit. In my youth the local bar was the substitute, still is. . . .Working class adults of my acquaintance were nearly all heavy and steady drinkers." The other, far more prevalent side of the picture, fits Cahalan's finding that the lower the "social index figure," the less likely a woman is to drink. Nancy Seifer, author of *Nobody Speaks for Me,* life histories of working-class women, says, "Of the ten women I interviewed and spent time with, only one had a drink, and she was the one whose husband had a drinking problem." Statistically, women who drink frequently are likely to have husbands who drink heavily, although the reverse is not necessarily so. True to cultural form, women seem more susceptible to social contagion.

The type of drink can be as revealing as the amount. Women as a group prefer sweet drinks and are less likely than men to drink beer, but beyond that generalization, you drink what you are, socially speaking. A *Vogue* reader with a college education and high income is likely to be comfortable with everything from hard liquor to wine to beer. In contrast to her wealthier, more eclectic sister, the middle-class woman usually sticks to ladylike sherry or wine and sweeter mixed drinks. The woman of working-class background who never went beyond high school is likely to drink beer or hard liquor if she does join the party.

A Long Island, New York, caterer (and caterers were chroniclers of taste long before social scientists even formulated their questionnaires) notes, "You can tell a lot about who and what people are by the things they want. Not long ago, there was an affair, a real society-page type of wedding, in an area where a lot of high-status old money lives. They ordered 250 double Old Fashioned glasses—we call them Texas jiggers. One of these very high-class affairs, where they give you plenty to drink [men's and women's drinking tastes converge more closely in this class than in others], but to eat, a piece of cheese on a cracker, not so much stress on food. At other affairs, they emphasize the food but order two kinds of wine glasses to let you know you're at a tasteful event."

Wine sales are growing faster than those of any other alcoholic beverage, and Vincent Sardi of New York's famous theatrical restaurant reports, "People are drinking wine instead of saying 'I'll have a dry martini.' "

Marietta Tree, the jet-setting urban planner, had twenty-four guests at a top-of-the-social-scale dinner party and used thirty-six bottles of white wine and a half-bottle of vodka. Her experience is typical of the in-group. Vodka has moved to the top of the popularity list in hard liquors for both men and women, edging out gin. *Jobson's Liquor Handbook* for 1984 reports that sales of vodka grew each year between 1965 and 1974 at a phenomenal rate of 8 to 12 percent. They peaked in 1981 with a whopping 31.6 million cases consumed. By 1984, consumption had leveled off at a point close to this figure, and analysts were predicting that soon vodka sales would surpass the sales of all types of whiskey lumped together. Vodka's popularity is attributed to its special virtues: It is colorless, lower in alcohol content for those who are worried about their intake (80 proof as against the 86–100 proof of whiskey), mixes unobtrusively with juices and sodas, leaves almost no telltale odor on the breath, and has a reputation for being hangover-free.

The remarkable rise in the popularity of wines and the increasing sophistication in buying and serving them are also reflected in Mrs. Tree's menu. "Most people have carafes of wine on the table," she pointed out, "so having a drink before dinner isn't that important." In her circle, too, white wine is a popular apéritif. Growth has slowed a little, but continues in the 1980s.

Women buy most of the table wine sold today, partly because twenty-six states allow it on their grocery store shelves. Women are also becoming increasingly aware of vintages and types and have moved in on the world of wine experts, with half a dozen women now acknowledged leaders. They are also joining the ranks of the drink snobs. Although Russell Lynes, a social critic and long-time editor of *Harper's* magazine, was talking only about men, what he said in 1950 is now equally applicable to women: "The Drink Snobs ... insist that their whiskey be bonded; they know what proof it is, and they drink it neat or 'on the rocks'; their Scotch is 'V.O.' or 'V.V.O.'; their martinis are as dry as almost no vermouth can make them (in restaurants where they suspect the martinis may be somewhat amber in hue they order Gibsons and remove the onions), and they always nod at the waiter after looking at the date on a bottle of wine. . . .Some Drink Snobs take special pride in the amount they can consume and not show it; others take special pride in having a worse hangover than anybody ever had before."

The French champagne industry reports gleefully that Americans bought 40 percent more champagne in 1976 than in the previous year, popping the corks on four million bottles. A sign of sophistication perhaps, or evidence that there are more Americans who see themselves as members of an educated elite and have the money to spend on luxuries.

Since 1960, wine sales have more than doubled. It's important to remember, though, that the popular (and usually less expensive) jug wines are sugared to appeal to soda-pop tastes, so the shift is more toward drinking moderately with food than away from sweetness. For those joining the temperance trend, wine coolers—wine mixed with nonalcoholic products—have become popular, with sales skyrocketing 380 percent in 1984. Actually, for health reasons, expensive wines (which usually contain no added sugar) are better for you—and, paradoxically, so is cheap liquor. It has been aged less and is therefore less likely to contain injurious tars and resins absorbed from those famous casks.

The rise in wine consumption isn't confined to the wealthy international traveler. Since drinking styles filter down from the top to the bottom of the social ladder, many women who don't see themselves as part of the drinking population now accept wine as a food or a symbol of the good life. A suburban New York newspaper editor in her late twenties, says, "If someone has a glass of wine, I don't think of that as alcohol. If I have some, it doesn't seem that I'm drinking. It's a status thing to be able to order the right wine—knowing what's a good year. Wine and cheese have achieved the middle-class respectability of church fundraising affairs. We even run a wine article once a month on the women's page." The highest per capita wine consumption is found in New York state and California—both major producers.

Wine has moved from supermarket shelves to the ballpark in California. A law enacted in the 1970s legalized its sale at professional sporting events seating at least forty thousand fans, and the San Francisco Giants supply the juice of good cheer in 6.4-ounce bottles. "Hey, get your cold beer" is yielding to "Hey, get your cold rosé, white or red." In deference to American—and particularly female American—tastes, the domestic jug wines passed along the grandstand aisles have a generous lacing of sugar. As one San Francisco sports columnist commented, "A couple of glasses of that stuff and you've got three tooth cavities."

This penchant for sweet drinks has been characteristic of women's drinking for a long time. In a relic of the days before "sex symbol" was a dirty phrase, *Esquire* magazine's 1948 Liquor Intelligencer (which did not even mention vodka) listed these women's favorites and their uses: "Pink Lady will put the lady in the mood for romance, of course. . . .Dancing is an easy transition; slow music. Suggest a Sherry Flip or, if thirsty, Cuba Libres under the umbrella."

Today, *Esquire*'s gimmicky drinks have virtually disappeared, to be replaced by other sweet summer fashions that may speed up the *seductio ad absurdum* of the magazine's earlier suggestions: a currently stylish frozen Daiquiri or Piña Colada has twice as much alcohol as the standard ounce-and-a-half jigger provides for less chichi mixed drinks.

Manufacturers counted on the female tendency to prefer smooth drinks when they marketed "pop" wines, such as Boone Farms—and pseudo-milk shakes, such as Malcolm Hereford's Cows. Market surveys had shown that these would sell best to young people, blacks, and women. Advertising, obviously designed to entice nondrinkers, emphasized taste rather than conviviality. Kickers, one of the flavored premixed drinks aimed at young people, was withdrawn from the market after complaints by the National Council on Alcoholism. Hereford's Cows was embroiled in a minor-league barroom brawl after consumer affairs expert Betty

Furness taped a TV segment showing twelve- to fourteen-year-old boys and girls drinking the strawberry-flavored stuff, which is 15 percent alcohol. She was, she says, trying to expose the way liquor companies go after young people, but she was reprimanded for serving alcohol to minors. In response to the criticism, Heublein, Inc., the manufacturer, said the sweet, creamy drink was designed, not for teen-agers, but for "middle-aged women." Because these new drinks don't fit into old patterns (beer is for men, sherry is for ladies), and there are no clear guidelines on quantity, they tend to be used and abused by inexperienced drinkers.

Another gimmick—powdered alcohol—is also outside established drinking habits. Developed by the Japanese and not yet on the world market, this product has liquid alcohol suspended in microscopic gelatine capsules. Premixed Bloody Mary's and screwdrivers in individual foil-wrapped packages need only water. Like other new ways of packaging alcohol, these "dry" drinks may help erase the differences in consumption between men and women.

The female sweet tooth has been remarked with some despair by the beer industry. "Women have definite reactions to taste differences, and tend to be less responsive to beer than men after their first experience with the beverage," an industry-wide study lamented. A stockbroker reinforces that conclusion: "I'm probably the only girl who got through four years of college without drinking beer. After one taste, I couldn't get the stuff past my lips."

Men are almost three times more likely to drink beer than women are. Women tend to drink it at home rather than in bars or taverns. Younger women are more likely to enjoy a stein now and then, but as incomes rise, the proportion of beer drinkers goes down as fast as a head of foam. Although beer is not identified as a blue-collar drink as much as it used to be, it is still not high-class enough to be offered on dressy occasions, and women who drink it usually do so in the company of men. (If women reject beer, the beer also rejects them. Foam sinks faster when a woman drinks because the grease in her lipstick deflates it.)

There are factors other than taste and working-class associations that keep beer from attaining what the brewing industry feels is its rightful place in feminine drinking habits. First, as the American Can Company reports regretfully, "It appears that girls have had sufficient experience with hard liquor to know their limitations but are not certain of their capacity for beer. They entertain the idea that, while a drink of hard liquor is sipped and nursed along, beer seems to slip down easily and could get out of hand." This cautious female attitude provided the Oklahoma legislature with an excuse for setting eighteen as the age when the obviously more sensible women could buy 3.2 beer, but twenty-one as the age for reckless young men. Women, the legislators claimed, were less likely to drive and get into auto accidents after drinking. In a landmark equal-rights decision, the U.S. Supreme Court in 1976[7] defended the men and said the law had to apply to both sexes equally.

In addition to inexperience and caution, there's another deterrent to women drinking beer—the calorie count. Beer has about 150 calories per twelve ounces, as against 100 for one and a half ounces (the usual jigger) of hard liquor. To cash in on the weight-watching obsession of both men and women, American brewers launched a massive campaign to sell what they call "light beer"—one-third lower in calories, high in taste. Within two years, it captured a sizable 4 percent of the market. On television alone, $84 million was spent in one year to push the new beverage. One commercial showed actor James Coburn saying, in a manly, threatening manner, "Schlitz Lite." That's all. This ad, said the creative director of the advertising agency, "appeals to both men and women, even though only a man appears."

The role advertising plays in affecting women's tastes is difficult to measure. Media experts point out that advertising doesn't create demand, it just makes it possible to profit from the demand that already exists. Even without advertising, people drink; in Russia, which has been without liquor ads for more than sixty years, vodka is still a best seller. It's generally agreed, though, that advertising does establish brand preferences, and that's where the competition comes in. With women—relatively innocent about brands—moving into prominence as drinkers, they have also moved into prominence on camera. First they appeared as smiling background figures in ads for wine, beer, and liquor. Then an attractive woman moved to the foreground, still smiling, but not obviously partaking. Now, women pour the wine, lift foaming glasses of beer, and sit holding the career woman's favorite—Scotch on the rocks. Industry guidelines have kept advertisers from going all the way; women (or men) are not to be shown actually drinking in print or on TV. Despite this restriction, the National Council on Alcoholism estimates that $750 million was spent to advertise beer and wine in 1984.

The stakes are high, with women almost half of the drinking force, and they must be convinced that brand X is better than brand Y. As one cynic observed, "People smoke cigar bands and drink labels." The educated taste is a myth—or at least something that very few people possess. As an industry summary reports, "blind taste-tests have repeatedly shown . . . flavor associations are psychological and in large part disappear when the brand label is removed from the product. They seem to be play-backs of imagery created by advertising." To test this, a shipbuilding magnate re-filled bottles of elegant Haig and Haig pinchbottle with inexpensive "Wee Burn Scotch Type" whiskey. Over a period of five years, only one of the fifty-four sophisticated friends who drank the liquor was able to guess it wasn't the real thing. The look of the bottle, not its contents, was what counted. With women now coming into the market at a faster pace then men, its not surprising that manufacturers are tailoring claims for their brands to appeal to feminine tastes, suggesting sexual as well as social advantages for their products. The industry has extra time to work; women's brand and drink preferences don't become firmly established as early as men's, often not until after marriage.

Despite the statistical reality that most Americans, men and women, drink moderately by any definition, a 1967 survey showed that when consumption was divided by number of drinkers the average user downed a whopping 815 drinks a year—more than two a day. By 1981, the total was just under 2.8 gallons of alcohol per year for every person fourteen years of age or older. Hardly a drop in the bucket compared to the hard-drinking days at the start of the nineteenth century when Americans drank an astonishing 7.1 gallons a person, but still considerable. Before the quibblers begin equating "average" with "moderate," it's well to remember that in real life rather than the never-never land of statistics, half of the alcohol is consumed by a minuscule 10 percent of the population—the heavy drinkers. When Dr. Cahalan did his study, about 75 percent of all Americans felt that alcohol does more harm than good, with, understandably, more women than men coming down on the negative side. In 1982, a Gallup poll showed that an overwhelming 81 percent of the population considered alcohol abuse a major national problem.

For young people, drinking is not so much a return to the freedoms of childhood, as Dr. Gomberg suggested, as it is a symbol of adulthood. Dr. Chafetz points out, "Our society doesn't have many rites of passage. There's no clear way to mark the change from being a child to being a grownup—except by doing what adults do—drink alcohol." Although the age at which youngsters reported their first drink used to be fourteen, it has now dropped to eleven—a precocious start on adulthood.

J. V. Rachal's national study of adolescent drinking behavior revealed in 1979 that 86.51 percent of all high school girls said they had tried alcohol. This was a low 25 percent as recently as fifteen years ago.

That rush to the bottle seems to be slowing down. The latest federal report on drinking shows that, although teen-age drinking is still a widespread problem, there is some evidence of a slight drop. What is clear—and has been since the late sixties—is that girls are catching up to boys in the percentage of them that drink. There is now very little difference between a young man and a young woman. In Orange County, California, a survey by Tom Alibrandi and Douglas Chalmers in the mid-1970s showed that 71 percent of the male and 65 percent of the female high school students drank—and the 6 percent gap continues to narrow. San Mateo County, California, has kept an eye on alcohol and drug use among its students since 1968; there, too, almost as many girls as boys report using alcohol, although they tend to drink less and to drink fewer times a month. But the number of girls who say they drink more than fifty times a year has tripled since 1970. The number of boys who do this has merely doubled. Nationally, 91.6 percent of all high school senior girls report they have used alcohol, a figure uncomfortably close to the 93.5 percent of boys.

One group has actually resisted the trend toward convergence of boys' and girls' drinking. The nationwide survey of teen-agers shows Hispanic girls to have the largest number of abstainers and the lowest consumption rate. Unlike their Anglo contemporaries, both Hispanic boys and girls still feel overwhelmingly that it is worse for a girl to drink.

And a wide-ranging look at drinking on thirteen college campuses across the country by Dr. Ruth C. Engs of the University of

Indiana shows that drinking problems among college students haven't increased dramatically in the past twenty-five years. What has changed is the amount of attention focused on drinking, and the fact that women are now drinking more—and the drink is hard liquor.

Contrary to another popular belief, the youngsters who use marijuana don't choose it in place of alcohol. They tend to use both, with one drug enhancing the effects of the other. Robert Pandina of the Rutgers Center of Alcohol Studies found that, in a New Jersey blue-collar community, the first use of alcohol coincided with the first use of marijuana at the surprisingly early age of twelve or thirteen.

In light of this disturbing picture, Dr. Ernest Noble, a spokesman on alcohol problems, said in 1977, "We now have American teen-agers who drink one or two times a week, with three to six drinks on occasion. These figures are based on children in school. What I wonder about are the dropouts, the runaways, the institutionalized children. We know nothing about them."

Family attitudes play a significant role in the drinking patterns of young people. Dr. Robert A. Zucker, professor of psychiatry at Michigan State University, found that "where parents agree and also have similar drinking patterns and attitudes, their children tend to follow that pattern, whether it be one of heavier drinking, moderate drinking, or abstention. . . .Where parents disagree, the outcome is also more complex; a disproportionate number are more likely also to develop later drinking problems." Surprisingly, even when parents agree about strict abstention from liquor, the children may have a higher risk of problems; maybe the unbending moral view forbidding drinking pushes some of them into rebellion and then guilt, which just intensifies the drinking.

For girls, the first drink is likely to be at home, prefaced solemnly with something like, "Now you're growing up and I want you to know what this stuff does to you before you head out on your own." Understood by both parent and child is the implicit message, "It's dangerous for girls to drink too much. Chastity and alcohol don't mix." Because of this emotional coloring, more women than men can remember their first drink. For the boys, the introduction often comes outside the house, with friends. Even for girls, though, the pressure to be "one of the gang" may provide the push toward adult patterns.

In some ways, teen-agers are moving faster than adults. The number of youngsters who have become drunk has more than doubled in the past twenty years and the National Institute on Alcohol Abuse and Alcoholism estimated in 1980 that a startling 3.5 million youngsters aged fourteen to seventeen were alcoholics or problem drinkers.

Concern about the epidemic is echoed by Douglas Chalmers, director of the alcohol-abuse program in the schools of Orange County, California. "What we have," he reported in a study of his students' drinking patterns, "is a pool of potential problem drinkers. They are disabled in the style in which they drink by the time they are in junior high school. Over 80 percent of our fourteen- and fifteen-year-olds have had a drink, and of the youngsters who drank more than once a month, 45 percent were heavy drinkers. Only 20 percent of our adult drinkers fit this category." Tom Alibrandi says sadly that when he gave a talk to a fourth-grade class of nine- and ten-year-olds at 9 A. M., two had already had a drink before school.

How do they get the alcohol? Some of them, of course, take it from home. At a suburban junior high school dance the boys and girls got drunk in the parking lot on a mixed hodgepodge of liquor they had been able to sneak from their parents' supplies without being caught. One mother was called to school that night to pick up her daughter. She found her in the bathroom, pale and penitent, throwing up. "Most of the parents are worried about drugs," the exhausted teacher on duty said. "I'm a lot more worried about alcohol. It's not just the boys—the girls are getting drunk, too." Other youngsters report they have very little trouble getting older teen-agers (of legal drinking age) or adults to buy beer for them in supermarkets, or wine or distilled spirits in a liquor store. They call it "pimping booze." Young women are more likely to drink beer than older ones—even if they are under age, it's easy to get. In a newspaper interview Kari, now seventeen, recalled: "My friends were all drinking beer when I was thirteen. They used to get it from older brothers and sisters, and they were always getting drunk."

Does this early pattern mean we can look forward to a rise in the number of alcoholics in the future? Dr. Patricia O'Gorman, co-author of *Teaching Alcohol*, a textbook for teachers, is concerned: "Every study shows that kids today are drinking younger.

What everyone is wondering is whether—since youth as a whole is drinking younger—this means we are going to have more alcoholics in twenty years. We just don't know."

What we do know from the Cahalan report is that "early drinking appears to be related to a tendency toward later heavy drinking." But even this ominous finding is tempered by the fact that this pattern appeared in men, and not in women. Girls who start drinking early don't necessarily become problem drinkers later and, since they are almost half the early drinking population, their pattern may take the edge off the dire predictions.

There's another reality. Dr. Kaye Fillmore, a sociologist who has followed teen-agers into adulthood with an eye on their drinking, says reassuringly: "Adolescence has traditionally been a time of freedom and experimentation. Just because a girl gets drunk and in an automobile accident—she may even kill someone—doesn't mean she's going to grow up to be alcoholic. If every teen-ager with drinking problems held onto that early pattern we wouldn't be studying alcoholics—we'd be studying that rare breed, the social drinker. The truth is most adolescents leave their excesses behind and grow up to drink with moderation."

Society tries, in various ways, to encourage this moderation. One is by establishing a minimum drinking age. Maimonides, the twelfth-century Spanish Jewish philosopher, suggested twenty-one as suitable, and his ancient wisdom has been adopted by many states. When Michigan lowered its drinking age to eighteen, there was an alarming increase in fatal automobile accidents involving teen-agers. Other states have not had the same horrendous aftermath, but many states, prodded by Mothers Against Drunk Driving (MADD), accident rates, and the threat of losing federal highway funds, have now raised the drinking age to twenty-one.

Dr. Charles L. Winek, editor of the *Toxicology Newsletter*, sees another difficulty. "My personal view," he says, "is that lowering the age to eighteen also carries with it a lowering of the 'challenge age'—that is, an increase in drinking among fourteen- to seventeen-year-olds because 'if eighteen-year-olds can drink why can't I?' or 'it's illegal to drink until you're eighteen so if I can get served I'll be on an ego trip.' The problem will never be solved by legislation. It's a human-behavior problem that must be solved at the family level."

With the bitter legacy of the twenties in trying to legislate morality still fresh, no one is suggesting that Prohibition is the way to stem the rising tide of new drinkers among teen-agers and women. Dr. Sheila Blume says tartly, "You can't ban something anyone can make at home. It's just too easy to produce." But alcohol abuse is also too pervasive a problem to be dumped in the lap of the family without some changes in society at large. There are a variety of possibilities. Sweden, with a hard-drinking population and a high proportion of alcoholics, earmarks 10 percent of its alcohol excise taxes to fight alcoholism. It also prints a health warning on every bottle of liquor, the equivalent of our "Smoking is dangerous to your health."

This country bases its federal excise taxes on the proof (or alcohol content) of the liquor, a policy that may account for the fact that some whiskeys have gradually lowered proofs to close to vodka's 80 instead of the traditional 86–100. This makes the drink less potent and gives the manufacturer more of the buyer's money, assuming that he keeps the price the same.

Canada's alarm at the increase in drinking and drinking problems prompted H. David Archibald, of Ontario's Addiction Research Foundation to make these suggestions: "We can control the number and types of outlets as well as the days and hours of sale. We can control the age at which alcohol is bought and consumed. We can certainly regulate the means by which alcoholic beverages are advertised and marketed, and we can manipulate the level of taxation which reflects on the overall cost of alcohol in the marketplace." England has recently found that taxes do cut consumption; Scotch is now taxed and priced out of the reach of many of its native drinkers. And English television networks have agreed to ban drinking on the home screen unless it is a necessary part of the story or documentary.

These sound like reasonable suggestions, but any attempts to regulate the liquor traffic—and people's drinking habits—run into two ineluctable obstacles: the commitment to freedom of choice (I have the right to decide whether, what, and how much I drink, even if it kills me) and the astounding economic reality that (according to the Distilled Spirits Council) federal excise taxes on alcoholic beverages rank fourth, after corporate and individual income taxes and the "windfall" profits tax on oil, as a source of revenue for the federal government. The more drinkers, the more dollars.

With millions of women now in the drinking force, and more joining it every day, it's not surprising that there has been a concerted effort to entice the second sex and keep consumption high. The right to drink, like the right to work outside the home, has become a mark of the liberated woman. But true liberation will come, as the director of a halfway house for alcoholics points out, when "in this society, it's also okay *not* to drink."

3

Effects on Body and Brain

*I*t's hard to imagine the history of the world without alcohol. It has been an integral part of religion and wars, of commerce and communion since civilization began. Even science owes fundamental advances to its importance—Pasteur developed the germ theory of disease while studying the fermentation of beer and wine; the process of making beer out of barley led to an understanding of the problems of gas pressure; and basic knowledge has come from chemists and microbiologists trying to unlock the structure of starch, the function of enzymes, and the role of yeasts and bacteria.

Yet alcohol itself remains a mystery. Probably the drug longest used by man, very little is known about precisely what it does in the body. No one yet understands how it causes intoxication or a hangover. Neurologists are still trying to find out exactly how it interferes with memory; and only very recently was it documented that alcohol itself—and not malnutrition—causes some of the physical damage noticed in most major body systems, from the liver to the heart to the brain. Long-term heavy drinking has also been implicated in processes that age the skin, dim the eyes, and dull the hearing.

Ethanol—C_2H_5OH, as it is known technically—is remarkable in other ways. Easily soluble in water, it invades every cell, every organ, every body system, and can affect every level of human activity. Unlike other foods, it doesn't have to be digested. It is absorbed directly from the stomach and small intestine into the bloodstream. Some of the absorption starts the instant alcohol lands in the mouth, with a small amount penetrating the mucous membrane. This speed is one of the things that has made drinking so popular—it works, and it works fast. Again, unlike other foods, alcohol can't be burned up by exercise. Only time and the liver, where most of it is metabolized, can get rid of it.

An ounce of 90-proof liquor has about seventy-five calories—the equivalent of five teaspoons of sugar—but they are empty calories, without other food value (except for some elements in beer and wine) and without vitamins. What they do is let the body store other calories as fat, so that optimists who point out that alcohol's calories can't be stored are forgetting that the body will then pad itself with calories from other food sources, which are not "extras."

How much alcohol gets into the bloodstream, and how fast, depends on a variety of factors. Someone who drinks one drink slowly, and takes an hour to do it, will probably match the body's ability to get rid of the liquor and will have no measurable alcohol in her blood at the end of that time. Someone who tosses down Scotch and water fast will have a higher blood-alcohol level than if the same drink had been consumed in three installments. There is an exception to the usual rule that slow drinking means slow absorption of the alcohol. In some sensitive drinkers, a quick slug of whiskey will be so irritating that the pyloric valve, between the stomach and the intestines, shuts tight in protest. This effectively keeps the liquor from moving into the bloodstream at its usual rate.

A full stomach slows the rate of alcohol absorption. An empty stomach gives the drug clear sailing into the intestines and then into the bloodstream. But contrary to fervently held convictions, no food is any more effective than any other in blocking the absorption of alcohol—not milk or caviar, or a few slugs of olive oil to line the stomach. This doesn't mean that the kind of food makes no difference. Since what is in the stomach before the alcohol gets there is what counts, slow-to-digest proteins and fats stay around longer and provide longer (although not necessarily better) protection. That's why the advice "Drink a glass of milk with a couple of egg whites in it before a cocktail party" is sound—the concoction is high in protein. Researchers who ask their subjects to fast for four hours so they can test alcohol's effects on an empty stomach have been stymied by pork products. "Some good fat spareribs the night before can really mess up our early-morning results. They seem to settle in the stomach forever."

Since alcohol's effects are directly related to weight, a 200-pound woman may be able to drink twice as much as one who weighs 100 pounds and get the same effect. Someone who's been able to handle two drinks without difficulty may suddenly discover that more than one makes her giggly. It could be that she's recently lost twenty pounds and should adjust her intake accordingly. Dieting can have other effects. Dr. J. Murray McLaughlan and his associates in Canada found that a healthy person who diets strenuously for even two or three days can become dangerously drunk on a few drinks.[1] Dieting cuts down on carbohydrates and so does alcohol. This can lead to a dramatic drop in blood sugar—hypoglycemia. Even though their blood-alcohol levels were low, the dieters felt and acted intoxicated.

Alcohol seems to be a stimulant. A little raises the spirits, but a lot reveals the drug for what it is, a central nervous system depressant which, like barbiturates, can lead to coma and even death. In small doses, it usually does what it is expected to do: make the shy person friendly, the hostile one pleasant, and the sad one happy. But studies of medical students at the University of Oklahoma by Dr. Ben Morgan Jones confirm what other scientists have guessed. Extroverts—outgoing, life-of-the-party types—are more affected by alcohol's depressant effects than introverts. This fits the cocktail party observation that the normally expansive, cheerful drinker may turn nasty after a while, but the quiet girl just gets a little less shy. The experimenters sorted the two personality types by psychological tests, then gave half of each group enough alcohol to reach intoxication. In the students who didn't drink, the extroverts did better on memory tests than the introverts. But among the drinkers, results were just the opposite. Alcohol slowed the extroverts more than it did their quieter classmates.

There is now some scientific evidence that the hallowed custom of drinking in the evening may have developed because that's the time the body is best able to adapt to alcohol. Studies at the University of Minnesota and the University of Arkansas show that susceptibility to alcohol is higher in the morning and early afternoon than in the evening, possibly because there may be a difference in the levels of liver enzymes that break down the drug. Food in the stomach from breakfast and lunch may also make a difference. In the Oklahoma laboratory, researchers found that subjects did worse on certain nonverbal psychological tests in the afternoon than in the evening, although people tested without alcohol were at their best earlier in the day. Of course, this may have something to do with expectation and previous drinking experience, both powerful influences. Most people have learned to handle alcohol's effects in the evening, when they are accustomed to drinking, but may not be so skillful earlier in the day.

Drinking in a tense, uncomfortable atmosphere or when anxious or depressed may intensify the action of alcohol. Dr. Morris Chafetz says, "If I had to come up with an unhealthy drinking situation, it would be the American cocktail party. Standing around uncomfortably in a crush of people, most of whom we don't know, makes us want to gulp that first drink."

Dr. Chafetz adds: "The way you drink is extremely important. You should always sip slowly. . . . Gulping alcohol produces a sudden, marked rise in the alcohol level in the blood and in the brain. Even if subsequent drinks are taken slowly, you will tend to have an unusually strong reaction to the dose."

Beer and ale are 3–6 percent alcohol; wine is 12–14 percent (but dessert wines, such as port and sherry, are 17–21 percent), and hard liquor is 40–50 percent. This is usually expressed as "proof"—80-proof whiskey being 40 percent alcohol by volume. In seventeenth-century England, alcohol content was estimated by dampening gunpowder with the beverage, and then lighting it. If the powder burned with a steady flame it was "proof" that the liquor was potent stuff—about 57 percent alcohol. In the United States, "proof" expresses double the alcohol content; in England and Canada, liquor that is 57.35 percent alcohol is "proof spirits." Anything below that is "under proof."

Although it's hard to believe, a twelve-ounce can of beer, a five-ounce glass of regular wine, and a one-and-a-half-ounce shot of whiskey have the same alcohol content. A drink is a drink is a drink. But tests reported by pharmacologists Chauncey D. Leake and Milton Silverman have shown that even when the beverages are consumed over the same time period, they produce different blood-alcohol levels because they are absorbed at different rates. Gin or whiskey on an empty stomach shoots the peak way up, dessert wines are next, and table wine and beer fall considerably lower. Two hours after the initial jolt, though, the levels are about the same.

This may explain the popularity of the martini which, swallowed before lunch or dinner, peaks high and fast. A quick drink is more potent than a slow one; gulpers absorb alcohol faster than sippers. This may be why alcoholics are likely to be gulpers and to prefer straight drinks. Champagne and drinks made with bubbly mixers are also transported more quickly into the bloodstream; the carbon dioxide (CO_2) speeds the process.

There are other things in liquor, wine, and beer besides alcohol and CO_2. These are called congeners—substances either added or naturally present which add taste and color and may affect the way a person reacts. One experimenter produced raging hangovers in people who thought they were drinking liquor when they were only drinking congeners. Fusel oil, one of the most common congeners, is used commercially as a lacquer solvent. A result of incomplete distillation, it causes thirst and headache in small doses. In large quantities, it is lethal. Beer, which used to be fairly innocent, is now doctored with additives such as gum arabic, as a stabilizer, and tannin, used to remove sediment. They improve the looks of the drink, but no one is sure what they do to the drinker. Vodka has the fewest congeners of any alcoholic beverage, and if it has been filtered over charcoal, it has none at all. Red wine, particularly the French variety, has a high tannin content and may increase the chances of stomach cancer in regular drinkers.

Alcohol reaches a peak in the bloodstream, then declines, and the up-curve feels different from the down-curve, even though blood-alcohol levels may be the same. Dr. Ben Morgan Jones looked into this aspect of drinking and commented: "It goes without saying that the amount of alcohol in your blood is the crucial factor. But important also is the stage of your blood-alcohol curve. In other words, are you getting high or coming down? It makes a difference not only to how you feel but also how you act and perform. Halfway down, you may feel and act sober, but your motor reactions may still be impaired." In his experiments, the top of the curve was reached about forty-five minutes after starting a drink.

To confirm what any party-goer could have told him, Dr. Jones invited four couples who knew each other to his laboratory and gave them the equivalent of four drinks throughout an evening. Their behavior was videotaped and recorded. As the blood-alcohol level went up (it was monitored periodically by having the participants blow into a Breathalyser), everyone became talkative and loud. They played Twenty Questions and charades and had a great time. After the curve started coming down (a yawn was the universal signal), people slowed down, slumped, and complained of being tired. Why this low feeling sets in is still open to question. The lateness of the hour may have had something to do with it. Dr. Jones also speculates that the start of the depression may impel people to take another drink and move their blood-alcohol level (BAL) into an up-curve again. He also notes that "animal studies show acetaldehyde [a product of alcohol metabolism] is higher in the brain when the BAL is increasing than decreasing. This may be one of the better explanations for what we've seen, since acetaldehyde has been implicated in the addiction process." To keep the acetaldehyde level high and avoid the unpleasant down-curve, a person reaches for another drink.

The most obvious, immediate effects of alcohol are on the brain. This pinkish gray organ, perched on top of the spinal column, is a double handful of tissue continually bombarded by electrical impulses. Its upper surface—80 percent of the whole—is a one-yard-long, two-foot-wide complex of cells folded and pleated to fit inside the unyielding skull of human beings. It is called the cortex, the center of thought, language, and abstraction, the crowning glory of the evolutionary process. Like the world, it is divided into two equal hemispheres, with the left side, in most people, controlling language, and the right side processing spatial perceptions and unconscious abilities. An older part, made up of an ancient cluster of glandlike structures and suborgans, controls the things we do without thinking—breathing, eating, sexual activity. One of these structures, the hippocampus, evidently is vital in the process of storing memories; when it is removed, patients remember what happened before the surgery, but can't retain for more than a few minutes anything that happens afterwards.

Despite recent prodigious steps forward in understanding the brain and how it works, researchers still know very little about how alcohol affects this three-pound control center. No one understands how drunkenness occurs, or how coordination is disturbed, or why memory is affected. One scientist laments, "There is more information available concerning biochemical processes associated with a variety of other centrally acting drugs than exists for a substance as ubiquitous and commonly used as ethanol."

That it is one of the mind changers is, of course, the chief reason for swallowing the stuff. But the changes are not always for the better, as Shakespeare recognized when he wrote, "Oh God! That men should put an enemy in their mouths to steal away their brains."

Traditionally, alcohol first steals away the part of the brain that has to do with judgment and restraint. After about two ounces of whiskey the drinker feels good—about herself, the world, and the future. This is at a blood level of 0.05. At the legal level of intoxication in many states—0.1—the motor areas of the brain become depressed. Speech flows less trippingly; the coat sleeve seems to move out of reach unexpectedly. Challenged, the drinker insists she is totally unaffected by liquor and often believes she can drive or rearrange her hair better than ever. A person who learns to monitor her own reactions can tell pretty well what her blood-alcohol level is as she approaches this point. First, she will feel warmth and a vague numbness in her cheeks and lips. Then her fingers, arms, and legs may tingle. As these start to feel numb, she is getting close to the 0.1 of legal intoxication.

At a 0.2 blood-alcohol level—five or more drinks in a short time—the midbrain is affected, producing unsteady gait and a tendency to feel better when lying down than standing up. At 0.3 the drinker can respond, but is in a stupor. A little more than that, and she goes into a coma, and at 0.6 or 0.7 the primitive, ancient centers that regulate breathing and heartbeat are disrupted, leading to death.

This is a neat "higher functions first—lower functions last" understanding of what alcohol does; the trouble is, it doesn't seem to be that clear-cut, although it certainly fits with observable behavior. More recent studies have shown that even at small doses, coordination may be affected before some of the so-called higher-center functions like memory, and that alcohol probably has some effect on all parts of the brain simultaneously.

It is, like ether, an anesthetic, dulling pain (and the sense of smell and hearing), but it is an unreliable surgical aid. So much is required to block out feeling that the patient runs the risk of having breathing and heartbeat stop abruptly. No wonder pioneering doctors were glad to switch to ether in place of whiskey when setting broken legs.

From a medical standpoint, drunkenness is alcohol poisoning. The slurred speech and weaving walk are evidence of overdose, not celebration. And the other changes that take place, such as a blunting of self-criticism and a feeling of freedom, may have more to do with culture than with cocktails. When Craig MacAndrew and Robert B. Edgerton of the University of California at Los Angeles (UCLA) looked at the way men and women in different societies act when under the influence, they found the drunk did whatever he was expected to do. If drunks in that culture were quiet, he was quiet. If they were wise, he was wise. If they ran after women, so did he. "In summary then," the researchers concluded, "when a spokesman for the conventional wisdom speaks of alcohol as (for example) 'the solvent of the superego' and, ipso facto, of the drunkard's comportment as 'a species of blind impulsivity,' he would do well to recognize the fact that he is dealing with a form of blindness that operates with its eyes open and with a species of impulsivity that possesses the peculiar ability to maintain a keen sense of the appropriate." What a person can get away with when drunk is, within certain neurological limits, what he or she has learned he can get away with. Alcohol gives the drinker a chance to say and do the things she's always wanted to, with society's permission, as long as that particular society's rules about how a drunk behaves are not violated.

It takes a lot more alcohol to produce drunken behavior in a person who has become accustomed to the drug. Like other addictive substances, alcohol makes it necessary to swallow higher and higher doses to achieve the same effect. What psychological or physical processes are involved in developing this tolerance are not yet understood. It is known that even an experienced alcoholic can swallow only twice as much as an abstainer before the action of the drug itself puts a stop to the guzzling. A morphine addict, on the other hand, can withstand a dose twenty to forty times higher than one that would kill a new user.

The phenomenon of tolerance can be a problem. Surgeons have recognized for years that alcoholics need more anesthesia and sedatives than other patients—their bodies have become accustomed to drugs. However, this is true only when they are sober. Drinking, they need less, because alcohol itself is an anesthetic.

Acquired tolerance may be only one part of the picture. Twin studies hint that there may be such a thing as inborn tolerance. Some people really seem to have been born with a hollow leg. Two scientists from the National Institutes of Health studied fraternal and identical twins and monitored their reactions to drugs, including alcohol. The fraternal twins varied as much as the general population in their responses. The identical twins, however, were strikingly similar—if one needed a lot to produce an effect, so did the other.[2] This is a clue that the ability to drink heavily may be genetic; so may the inability to tolerate much alcohol. People who can drink a lot may be congenitally more likely to develop alcohol problems than those who are protected against large amounts because drinking makes them feel awful.

Along with tolerance—the ability to handle larger and larger amounts of the drug—comes the other inevitable companion of addiction, withdrawal symptoms. Alcohol is an addictive drug because it produces both these effects. An alcoholic undergoing withdrawal (and this can happen when drinking stops abruptly, or even when the blood-alcohol level falls a minor amount) feels unbearably anxious, sweats profusely, shakes, throws up, and may even see things that aren't there and go into convulsions. In extreme cases the D.T.'s—"snakes are crawling all over me"—develop. Long a subject for inappropriate comedy, delirium tremens is fatal in a small percentage of cases even when everything medically possible has been done.

It is probably mild withdrawal symptoms that contribute to the curse of the social drinker, the hangover. The signs are unmistakable, although not everyone always has all of them: a head that feels like someone is hammering on it, a parched throat, and furry tongue. Trembling hands. A stomach whose churnings threaten periodically to erupt. The fervent wish that the sun would go away and hide. And the compelling impulse to hiss "shh" when the cat tiptoes across the room. How much of this is purely physical—the result of too much alcohol the night before—and how much psychological is still being debated.

Chances are slim that the question will ever be answered. Research on human beings is necessarily limited, and few animal models foolish enough to be voluntary fellow sufferers have yet been found. Scientists have tried. At the University of Oklahoma researchers used African guinea hogs, about the same weight as men, in the hope that they would be willing to overindulge. They had already shown that they share another human vice—overeating. Unfortunately, the only way they could be persuaded to accept alcohol was after exposure to the brutal summer sun for three days without water. Then they drank beer to drunkenness, developed the staggers, and seemed to lose their sense of fear (as many human beings do). The experiment ended abruptly, however, when the hogs who stubbornly remained teetotalers began to eat the tails of their inebriated relatives.

So much for attempts to study hangovers in animals. In people, there are four ways of looking at the misery: as the direct result of alcohol's irritant effects, as withdrawal symptoms, as fatigue, and as more psychological than physical.

Swallowing liquor is a little like swallowing sandpaper. When the alcohol hits the stomach, it irritates the sensitive lining and may even kill some of the cells. This is enough to explain the heartburn and indigestion of the morning after. Alcohol also dilates the blood vessels in the brain; the increased pressure causes headache, not only in the heavy drinker but in anyone who is subject to migraines or cluster headaches. The body's balance of water and salts is disturbed, too, forcing water out of the cells and into the spaces between. On top of that, the part of the brain that limits urination is dulled. That's why the drinker may get rid of more fluids than usual and feel desert-dry the next morning.

The shakes, nausea, and sensitivity to light and sound are really mild withdrawal symptoms—the second contributor to the misery—indicating that the body and brain had become accustomed to the drug and were acting up because it was no longer there. In the encyclopedic two-volume *Actions of Alcohol,* the authors state, "All the symptoms of hangover combine with hyperexcitability (extreme sensitivity) to define a state which resembles a mild abstinence syndrome." The ancient wisdom that another drink is the best cure for these miseries is evidence, they say, that the trouble is withdrawal. Like the morphine addict who is relieved of painful muscle cramps only by another shot, the hangover sufferer settles down after another drink. Striking color photographs in a medical magazine of a hangover sufferer's stomach vividly show the angry red subsiding to pink after a dose of alcohol.

Some experts are more inclined to feel that the hangover is the body's response to extreme fatigue, although they concede that alcohol itself can produce the same effects. The drinker pushes herself beyond her usual exhaustion level because alcohol dulls her awareness of how tired she is. The next day, the discomforts that descend are the body's way of signaling, "Sleep it off. Give me time to recover from my exertions."

Drinking in a tense situation can also contribute to fatigue. A morning-after drink helps the tense-and-tired hangover by once more dulling the exhaustion. But it is like fighting fire with fire and can get out of control. It only delays the real treatment, rest.

Another kind of hangover—the "sangria syndrome"—may hit the person who doesn't drink much at all. These sufferers eat all the fruit in the bottom of the pitcher, very little of the liquid, and wake up the next morning with a raging headache. As non-drinkers, they may have felt deep guilt pangs about what they were doing and were duly punished, not by their bodies so much as by their consciences. There's also the woman who feels there's a price for every pleasure—drink at night, suffer in the morning, even if the dosage isn't very high. Then, of course, there are the people who are peculiarly sensitive to small doses, physically rather than psychologically.

The part expectation plays in the cause and cure of hangovers has led to a book full of recipes for preventatives and remedies, ancient and modern. They all work, more or less, depending pretty much on the faith of the drinker. The Romans were assured, "If you wish to drink much at a banquet, before dinner dip the cabbage in vinegar and eat of it as much as you wish and likewise when you have dined, eat five leaves. The cabbage will make you as if you had had nothing and you can drink as much as you will." The Greeks had a word for hangover—"crapula." In attempting to relieve postbanquet headaches, they bound their foreheads tightly with celery or laurel or whatever else was around. These garlands soon became symbols of success; only the powerful could afford to have hangovers. The laurel wreath that began as a remedy soon became an accolade, as Arthur P. McKinlay explains in his article, "Bacchus as Health Giver."

Coffee is a more recent remedy. As a quick way to sober up, it is virtually useless. What you get is a wide-awake drunk. The same is true of a brisk walk around the block or a cold shower. For practical purposes, the only thing that burns up alcohol is the liver, and it refuses to be rushed. The next morning, though, coffee may do some good by helping the blood vessels in the head to shrink to normal size. On the other hand, the caffeine may also stimulate a person to get up and get going, encouraging still more fatigue at the final reckoning. The grim reality is that sleep and aspirin, if the protesting stomach can tolerate it, are the best remedies.

This truth hasn't interfered with the popularity of more exotic substances. Cures have involved prairie oysters (tomato juice, a raw egg as the "oyster," a dash of Worcestershire sauce, and salt and pepper); Bloody Marys (tomato juice and vodka), often offered at the start of Sunday brunch on the assumption that anyone worth inviting has been out the night before; and bullshots (consommé, lemon juice, Worcestershire sauce, Tabasco, and vodka). All these have one thing in common, vitamin C. It's possible that vitamin C is in some mysterious way involved in how alcohol affects the body. Rats predosed with it and then exposed to repeated injections of alcohol had lower blood-alcohol levels than the ones in an unprotected group.[3]

Most of the popular remedies for what the French call *gueule de bois* ("woody mouth") and the Swedes label *hont i haret* ("pain in the roots of the hair") probably depend more on what the patient expects than on what is in the concoction. In an experiment to test this theory, a nauseated patient was given a dose of syrup of ipecac, a classic drug for inducing vomiting in poisoning cases. The man, however, was assured that this was a superb potion that would calm his stomach immediately. It did, even when gastric activity was measured by scientific instruments.

Scientists have been searching for a sobering-up pill for years. It would speed the elimination of alcohol from the body and, if added to the bartender's wares, could prevent endless brawls and automobile accidents. It would also help avoid deaths from alcohol overdoses. Drinkers would not have to wait for time and the liver to do the job. The only thing that seems to work so far is intravenous infusions of fructose—fruit sugar—given in such massive doses that vomiting often results. The treatment can also be dangerous because it depletes the energy-transferring chemicals in the liver. Many drunks would rather take their chances with a hangover and choose to remain drunk. Some doctors suggest eating a lot of honey (on toast, for instance) after drinking, hoping that the fructose in the honey will do the trick. It probably won't.[4]

Other researchers are hunting for something that will block the deleterious effects of alcohol in the body. An alcoholic might then avoid further damage to her liver or heart while she struggled to control her drinking. In Canada there are experiments with a drug that blocks the euphoric effects of alcohol. If no "high" results from drinking, maybe people with problems will decide it's not worth the trouble.

Sophisticated instruments that measure sleep activity have confirmed conventional wisdom—a drink or two before bedtime speeds the coming of sleep, but, as with most benefits of alcohol, this one has a catch. The alcohol interferes with essential REM (rapid eye movement) or dreaming sleep, particularly in the first part of the night. Then, as it wears off, the body rushes to make up the dreaming time that has been lost, and the sleeper tosses and turns until morning. She has slept but not rested and wakes weary and irritable.

The steady drinker's body soon adjusts itself to this rebound effect—intriguing evidence that tolerance to the drug develops in the brain, affecting the electrical signals that can be recorded on an electroencephalograph. These tracings also show that although their dreaming may be spread out normally, chronic alcoholics have less deep, restful sleep than normal subjects, objective evidence of the insomnia and night terrors of which alcoholics often complain.[5]

Dr. B. K. Lester and his associates tried giving alcoholics small doses of alcohol and found that "the hair of the dog" miraculously normalized their sleep patterns, raising the fascinating possibility that some alcoholics really do cure their insomnia by drinking. Even after years of being "dry," people who have abused alcohol have trouble sleeping soundly. This is one of several indications that the drug or one of its by-products (particularly when associated with malnutrition or head injuries) actually leads to the death of brain cells in many alcoholics. CAT (computerized axial tomography) scan X-rays of heavy drinkers show shrunken brains. The brain ages prematurely (time, too, kills cells) and an alcoholic's brain waves often look like those of a person ten or fifteen years older. This grim possibility, a cornerstone of the early temperance movement, doesn't mean that "every drink kills cells." It does mean that alcohol may do permanent damage when consumed in large quantities. "It is becoming increasingly clear," writes respected researcher Dr. Alfonso Paredes, in a look at the direction future studies should take, "that the toxic effects of the drug on the brain persist long after the use of alcohol has been discontinued."

Even in small quantities, the drug affects memory, particularly of the short-term "telephone number" variety. Memory is the computerized library of the mind. An event or a fact has to be recorded, stored, and then retrieved, and interference with the process at any of these points is what we call forgetting. But just how the system works is still an enigma. If the process were a purely physical one, brains would have to be mountainous to contain all the information. Perhaps, scientists have speculated, memory is hidden in electrical circuits, laid down in specific parts of the brain, most likely the cortex. To check this out, Karl Lashley, a pioneering neuropsychologist, taught rats to run mazes, then cut out various parts of the cortex hoping that at some point he would also cut out the memory of what the rats had learned. No matter how much he cut, the memory persisted and the maimed rats, some staggering because of brain damage, dutifully did what they had been taught. Obviously, learning was more complicated than he had thought.

More recently the search has concentrated on chemicals in the brain which might explain why some memories survive head injuries, electric shock therapy for schizophrenia, and other conditions that play havoc with electrical currents. Could memory and protein be linked? As an unlikely understudy for human beings, researchers at the University of Michigan chose the goldfish. Credited with good memories (they are miniature relatives of the legendary carp who, once hooked, stays away from fishermen for the rest of its long life), the goldfish were taught to swim across a barrier in their pool. Ordinarily, they had no trouble remembering this for a month. Then Dr. Bernard Agranoff injected puromycin, a drug that interferes with protein production, into their brains right after they had been trained. The usually responsive fish acted as if they had never seen the signal light before. Evidently, the drug had kept them from recording what they had learned. If it hadn't been recorded, it couldn't be recalled, and the recording seemed to have something to do with proteins in the brain.[6]

It has been known for a long time that even moderate doses of alcohol interfere with short-term memory, and that women seem to be more vulnerable than men. Only recently has there come a hint that women social drinkers may do permanent damage to this kind of recall. More than a hundred women were tested before and after a drink on their ability to remember for a few minutes words that had been flashed on a screen. They all did worse after one drink, but moderate drinkers scored lower than light drinkers, with "moderate" defined by Bible Belt Oklahoma standards as one drink a week and "light" as one drink a month. When researchers Ben Morgan Jones and Marilyn K. Jones tried to figure out if age had anything to do with the fact that some women lost more memory than others after a drink, they discovered that "the young person who uses more alcohol behaves more like an older person who uses less alcohol. And the length of time a person has used alcohol is probably more important than age in memory loss. What scares me," Dr. Jones continues, "is what small doses of alcohol can do to your memory. We're talking about blood-alcohol levels of 0.04 or 0.05—0.1 is the usual legal definition of intoxication."

Dr. Jones is convinced alcohol and not marijuana or tranquilizers, for instance, interfered with memory. "Around here in Oklahoma," he pointed out, "it's a lot easier to say 'no other drugs complicated the tests' than it would be in California or New York. This is about as clean a sample of people as you can get in today's times."

What might be going on in the brain to cause words to fade almost as soon as they have been learned is still unknown. But Dr. Ernest Noble and his colleague Dr. Sujata Tewari reported that mice fed alcohol in concentrations roughly equivalent to wine every day for six weeks or more (in "social drinking" amounts) were not able to manufacture brain proteins at their usual rate. As in the puromycin-fed goldfish, brain-protein synthesis decreased in the alcohol-fed rats. Since proteins and memory seem to be related, this might explain alcohol's action.

Anyone who has ever gone to a cocktail party has noticed how people step on each other's words without waiting for a sentence to end. There's also a tendency for the second speaker to take off on her own subject, no matter what she thinks she's responding to. This phenomenon was subjected to scientific scrutiny at the University of California at Irvine where eighteen couples were plied with liquor and their conversations tape-recorded. After enough alcohol, they not only broke into each other's conversations but "seemed less likely to follow conventional rules of etiquette in their speech." [7] Some of this unseemly behavior may have been due to alcohol's expected effect on inhibitions in this society; but some of it may have resulted because the drinkers couldn't really remember what the other person was talking about. There's even the possibility that, since alcohol affects hearing when there is more than one noise to be accounted for, the hubbub cut down on what was heard as well as what was remembered.

In a curious reversal of its usual effects, drinking is sometimes credited with improving memory. If a person learns something—a word list, a poem—even when severely intoxicated, chances are it will be recalled more accurately drunk than sober. This is called state-dependent learning. It has some strange manifestations. Dr. Donald Goodwin of the University of Kansas Medical Center, tells the story of one of his patients, a forty-seven-year-old housewife who "often wrote letters when she was drinking. Sometimes she would jot down notes for a letter and start writing it but not finish it. The next day, sober, she would be unable to decipher the notes. Then she would start drinking again, and after a few drinks the meaning of the notes would become clear and she would resume writing the letter: 'It was like picking up the pencil where I had left off.' "

There is also the reverse effect on memory—amnesia ("Say, Alice, tell me. Did I do anything stupid at the party last night?"). The fearful morning-after phone call often signals an alcoholic blackout. These memory lapses have nothing to do with passing out and can hit social drinkers as well as alcoholics, but since they are triggered when the blood-alcohol level rises to a high point quickly, they are most often experienced by heavy drinkers. Alcohol experts divide blackouts into two kinds. The first is not really a complete blank. The drinker may be hazy about what she did, remember fragments, or remember only with prompting ("You're right. I did leave my shoes in the downstairs hall."). This phenomenon is sometimes called a "brownout." Often, the memory seems unreal, or as if it happened to someone else.

The second kind of blackout is a complete loss of any recall. It is really gone. Nothing can bring it back. According to Dr. Goodwin, who has made a study of memory and alcohol, no one knows just how this happens. But alcohol, he says, "in some people on some occasions [probably] interferes with chemical processes that make memory—perhaps the most mysterious of biological phenomena—possible." The use of other drugs, malnutrition, and head injuries may play a part, too. Inexplicably, someone in a blackout looks and acts fine, is able to travel, talk intelligently, and perform complex tasks. But whatever chemical step (perhaps connected with proteins) it is that turns short-term memories into long-term ones is obviously disrupted when a blackout occurs, and no amount of prodding can bring back what may have been recorded but never placed on "hold." One woman played tournament bridge—and won—although she couldn't remember laying a card on the table. A person will probably not do anything during a blackout that she wouldn't do when just plain drunk, but the inability to remember makes the gap seem filled with awful possibilities. An alcoholic woman patient of Washington, D.C., psychiatrist Benjamin Karpman told him, "It seems to me the blanks I experience when drinking are entirely governed by the amount of alcohol consumed. Up to a certain point in an evening, I can remember everything; then things become hazy and then totally gone as far as remembering is concerned. The things you imagine you did or are afraid you did may be much worse than the actual events, but it is the uncertainty of it that drives me crazy." Dr. LeClair Bissell, formerly of the Smithers Treatment Center in New York, says the ultimate horror is "for a woman to wake up in bed with a man she doesn't know." Heavy drinkers may soon have a choice about avoiding blackouts. Scientists at the National Institute of Alcoholism and Alcohol Abuse (NIAAA) gave the experimental drug Zimelidine to men before a heavy drinking episode and found the subjects avoided alcoholic blackouts. Some didn't feel this was an advantage, however, since "they were embarrassed because they remembered what they had done when they were drunk."

A history of blackouts has traditionally been used to diagnose alcoholism in the early stages, but when Dr. Jane E. James finally looked at women, she found amnesia occurred later in the downward spiral. As a symptom, it is more serious in a woman than in a man, but men are more likely to suffer this kind of memory loss, probably because they drink larger quantities.

A more crippling, pervasive kind of amnesia occurs in some chronic alcoholics. Called Wernicke-Korsakoff disease after the

German and the Russian who first described it, this kind of memory loss is probably due to a deficiency of vitamin B_1 (thiamine). If massive doses of the vitamin are not given early enough, permanent damage results and the alcoholic needs chronic care. The brain damage somehow affects immediate and short-term recall. Like the woman who puts her eyeglasses down and five minutes later can't find them, but clearly remembers her third-grade teacher, the sufferer from Wernicke-Korsakoff's syndrome may recall the past but draw a blank for what happened a few minutes ago.

More subtle kinds of brain damage are also associated with the use of alcohol. Whether it is the alcohol itself that assaults the little gray cells is still being debated, but it now seems that the right side of the brain is more vulnerable than the left. In split-brain experiments, scientists have discovered that the left side is involved with words, and the right with abstract reasoning and the ability to visualize things in space. When alcoholics were given vocabulary tests, they did just as well verbally as nonalcoholics with similar IQ's and education. When they were presented with a special set of cards and told to sort them according to color, form, and shape, then switch to another way of sorting them, they fell far behind. For one thing, they didn't distinguish as clearly which shapes went with which; for another, they had trouble shifting to a different way of looking at the same things.[8]

With these studies in mind, Elizabeth Parker, a psychologist at the University of California, and Ernest Noble, former head of the NIAAA, decided to see if social drinkers, too, were more affected on one side of the brain than the other. They evaluated more than a hundred suburban California men who were moderate or heavy social drinkers on the same kinds of tests at a time when they'd had nothing to drink for twenty-four hours. The results were astonishing. The men who reported they were moderate drinkers did better on the visual and spatial tests than the ones who said they were heavy drinkers. As the amount a man drank on each drinking occasion went up, his ability to deal with abstractions went down. There seemed to be no connection with how long a man had been a drinker; if he averaged five or six drinks at every party, he did poorly. The researchers aren't saying categorically that alcohol caused the differences. They recognize that life stresses or other factors may have made one group drink more and coincidentally perform more poorly than another. They do suggest, ominously, that research ought to be conducted on whether these deficits can be reversed. Is there a vitamin or other substance that will restore the right side of the brain to full functioning even if someone has been drinking moderately or heavily for years?

Evidence that even one drink can affect a person's ability to deal with spatial abstractions comes from a study by B. C. Chandler and Oscar Parsons, who have been particularly interested in how alcohol affects the brain. Compared with subjects who were given an orange drink with an alcohol "float" to fool them into thinking they were really getting a drink, the men who had the real thing took significantly longer to search for shapes on the left side of their field of vision. (For some mysterious reason, the right side of the brain controls the left hand.) These findings, although admittedly preliminary, are not comforting to business-lunch drinkers who may have to deal with tricky questions when they get back to the office. They may talk convincingly, but their ability to see things in broad perspective may not be at its best. And they may not even be conscious of their diminished ability.

Obvious physical brain damage has been estimated in 50–70 percent of chronic alcoholics. Now, with the space age technology that has produced CAT scans, doctors are getting a clear look at the cerebral atrophy without waiting for surgery or an autopsy. Combining the computer with X-rays, CAT gives three-dimensional pictures of soft tissue like the brain. For the first time, changes in soft tissue can be studied without subjecting the patient to sometimes hazardous injections of dye or air. Early studies by Dr. Phillip S. Epstein and his colleagues on a small number of patients at Presbyterian-St. Luke's Rush Medical Center in Chicago turned up the discouraging possibility that women may be more prone to this kind of damage than men. This may be because the women in this study, as in several others, were more likely to be periodic or "bender" drinkers, and high levels of alcohol maintained over a period of days seem to have harsher effects than slightly lower levels maintained over a longer time. The women with demonstrable brain damage were also twenty years younger than the men—between thirty and thirty-nine, rather than fifty and fifty-nine—another suggestion that women may be particularly sensitive.

The news is not all bad. One of the few pieces of evidence that a little alcohol may be a good thing comes out of the University of Michigan. As reported in *Newsweek* (August 26, 1974), researchers there tested students' ability to repeat words in Thai—a language none of them had ever heard before. One drink and anxiety went down; words remembered went up. More alcohol than that, though, and tongue and brain stopped cooperating. As a matter of fact, the volunteers were tested for intelligence along with language ability, and the latter went down steadily as the amount of liquor increased. Sadly, one of the psychologists concluded, "Alcohol has a distinct disadvantage if you have to use your brains."

What about alcohol enhancing creativity? Certainly many famous women writers have had reputations for hard drinking, the satirist Dorothy Parker and the poet Edna St. Vincent Millay among them. Scientists have always been skeptical that the juice of the grape helped the creative juices to flow, but they may soon start paying serious attention to the possibility. Drs. K. W. Wanberg and J. L. Horn of Denver, after studying 2,300 men and women, suggested that the recurring reports of improved performance after drinking couldn't be dismissed as misperceptions. "It is worth considering," they wrote, "that particularly in creative work, it may sometimes be desirable to lower inhibitions and standards in order to improve performance."

On the other hand, literary critic Alfred Kazin, who looked at the writing of several great drinkers who were also great writers, asserts that as alcohol consumption went up, the amount of good writing usually went down. Perhaps, as Sir William Osler, the great Canadian physician, remarked, "Alcohol does not make people do things better; it makes them less ashamed of doing them badly."

This is also true of drinking and driving. One woman said, "I always feel I can drive better after a few drinks even though I know it isn't true." After one drink, an *experienced* driver is no more likely to get into an accident than if she'd had nothing. After two drinks, she is twice as likely to get into trouble. An *inexperienced* driver may have trouble with even one drink—newly learned skills are the first to go. What alcohol does is affect a whole series of factors that are involved in complex physical skills. The ability to adjust to glare is reduced (so night driving becomes particularly tricky), reaction time is slowed, hand steadiness is decreased, and, most important of all, a person's ability to react to the unexpected is affected. This is especially true on the downward curve of the blood-alcohol level—the time in the evening when a drinker feels sober but has the same amount of alcohol in her blood as she did earlier, when she felt unmistakably high. "You may feel and act sober," Dr. Jones cautions, "but you can't do as well as you think you can. If any unusual thing happens—if a child runs out between parked cars—your reaction time would be slowed." Alcohol also affects the ability to detect sounds and slows reaction time to what is heard. Smoking adds to the dangerous possibility that a driver's hearing will be impaired.

According to the Department of Health and Human Services report on alcohol and health, a few drinks may also make a person underestimate the speed of objects and distance traveled, and may decrease fear, leading to reckless driving. Dr. Chafetz, generally inclined to look on the bright side of social drinking, warns, "Any drinking that begins to push our blood-alcohol level above the 0.05 mark impairs our driving. The higher the blood-alcohol level, the higher the risk." Frightening national statistics indicate that 50 percent of all drivers killed in highway accidents were legally "impaired." What this may mean, says Mark Goff, a young watchdog of alcohol programs in Milwaukee, is that, "since many of the people involved in fatal accidents weren't problem drinkers, probably the only problem they had with alcohol was that it killed them." To be on the safe side, Dr. E. M. Jellinek, acknowledged father of the field of alcohol studies, suggested, "If you take two ounces of whiskey, I'd say wait about one hour before you drive. If you take four ounces, wait two hours, and for each additional ounce, add one hour."

When alcohol enters the bloodstream, it triggers minor but pervasive chemical changes. One of them slows down the production of white blood cells, the body's defense against infection, making the chronic drinker susceptible to disease. Another may offer a way to diagnose alcoholism without relying on self-reporting or withdrawal symptoms or severe physical damage. Three doctors at the Bronx Veterans' Hospital in New York tested the blood of men hospitalized for alcoholism. They also drew samples from men hospitalized for other reasons. Even though the alcoholics were not drinking at the time, the doctors found a biochemical marker in their blood that wasn't present in the blood of the other patients. They continued to pick this up for as long as a week after drinking had stopped. Why this marker—an imbalance in amino acids, the body's building blocks—occurs is still being investigated. But Dr. Spencer Shaw and his colleagues, working in the laboratory of Dr. Charles Lieber, found it in well-nourished as well as malnourished long-term heavy drinkers, and were even able to duplicate the results with well-fed baboons. They hope their work will lead to a simple test that can identify alcoholics and get them into treatment before permanent physical damage occurs.

Like most other research, this involved only men. But there is no reason to believe it doesn't also apply to women. Alcohol's damaging effects are usually no respecter of sex. As Dr. Bernard Heyman, then at Grasslands Hospital in New York's Westchester County, told parents concerned about teen-age drinking, "Of all addictive agents, two are without question physically damaging and life threatening. These are the two legal ones—alcohol and tobacco." Like many substances, alcohol seems to be fairly harmless or even helpful in small quantities; in large ones it can be fatal. A suburban high school fraternity member chugalugged a pint of whiskey on a dare and was saved from certain death only by the quick action of a hospital emergency team. An Alfred University (New York) college student was not so lucky. He died after swallowing half a pint of whiskey as part of a fraternity initiation.

Less dramatically and more slowly, alcohol works chiefly on three areas of the body: the heart; the central nervous system, including the brain; and the digestive system, including the liver. As for the heart, the news is both good and bad. There is evidence that moderate drinking—one beer a day—may prevent heart attacks and even do as much as a low-fat diet in dissolving the plaques of fatty substances that clog arteries and predispose one to coronary occlusion. Even abstainers had more heart attacks than the drink-a-day subjects. These reassuring results from a study by Dr. Katsuhiko Yano and his associates on more than seven thousand men of Japanese ancestry living in Honolulu was greeted by the medical establishment with a joyful editorial in the staid *New England Journal of Medicine:* "Although one does not want to make too much of the apparent benefits, what data there are show, if anything, a lower incidence [of heart attacks] in those who drink a little. . . . It is encouraging to note that not everything one enjoys in life predisposes to cardiovascular disease. There is nothing to suggest, for the present, that we must give up either coffee or alcohol in moderation to avoid a heart attack. I am sure that many who read this editorial will be quite willing to drink to that statement." Since that early gleeful assessment, evidence has accumulated that moderate drinkers—both men and women—live longer than nondrinkers and heavy drinkers and have lower rates of heart attacks. A little alcohol increases the body's store of high-density lipoproteins, organic compounds formed from lipids and proteins that some researchers feel are a protective factor against heart disease.[9]

Other physicians are quick to point out that the chronic drinking of large amounts is another matter. Dr. G. Douglass Talbott, reporting at a National Council on Alcoholism scientific conference, warned, "Present evidence indicates that the heart may be the organ [of the body] most dangerously affected." Even a normal heart, he points out, can be so injured that it can't do its job efficiently. Here's how one alcoholic woman remembers her frightening experience: "I thought I had the flu, or it was the pollution, or I was jogging too much. I just couldn't catch my breath. Finally the only way I could sleep was propped up on three pillows. The third doctor I went to recognized it for what it was: alcoholic cardiomyopathy. My lungs were filling with fluid because my heart muscle wasn't working right, and I could have died any time. Luckily it scared me into stopping drinking, and I haven't had any more trouble." Obligingly, once the assault from alcohol stops, the heart gradually repairs itself—unless overwhelming damage has occurred.

There is new evidence, based on the work of Dr. Charles Lieber, that alcohol itself, and not the traditional villain, malnutrition, does the harm. Dr. Emanuel Rubin, former chief of pathology at Mount Sinai School of Medicine in New York, thinks that alcohol's effect on calcium in the body may explain what happens to muscles in general, not only the heart muscle. He told Arthur Fisher, a *New York Times Magazine* writer, "Recently we performed some tests on a heart muscle, in a test tube. . . . We know that one of the key elements in the contraction and relaxation of heart muscles— or any skeletal muscle—is the capture and release of calcium by certain parts of the muscle cell. We have found that alcohol interferes significantly with this ebb and flow of calcium."

The muscle weakness associated with alcoholism doesn't end

with the heart; it has been noticed for 150 years in other parts of the body. Healthy subjects at Mount Sinai were required to drink about a fifth of whiskey a week for four weeks. When samples of their muscles were looked at under the electron microscope, severe damage was revealed. Like the woman with heart damage, however, everything returned to normal after six months away from heavy drinking.

The chance that small amounts of alcohol can damage the heart muscle was demonstrated by Dr. Leigh Segal of the University of California at Davis. Using man's customary stand-in, the rat, she produced heart-muscle damage after seven weeks even with moderate doses—the equivalent of two cocktails a night. Higher doses produced not only microscopic changes, but disturbances in the way the heart worked.

Muscle weakness of another kind, produced by damage to nerve fibers which control the muscles of the legs, is sometimes a complication of severe alcoholism. An athletic-looking alcoholism counselor, who now strides easily along hiking trails as a dedicated bird watcher, remembers her bout with this crippling side effect—peripheral neuropathy. "I was forty-four years old. I holed up in my apartment with cases of booze and drank without eating until I weighed seventy-eight pounds. My legs were so weak I couldn't walk. They found me and put me in the hospital for nineteen weeks, and then released me with braces on both my legs. For some God-awful reason that I'll never understand, when I was dropped off at a friend's apartment I didn't go inside. I struggled three blocks to the nearest liquor store." It took another round in the hospital and then time in an alcoholism treatment center before she was able to give up alcohol and regain her health. Her legs are now fine, although not everyone is so fortunate.

The remarkable ability of the body to regenerate itself given some "dry time" away from alcohol is nowhere more staggeringly evident than in the liver, where 90 percent of the alcohol consumed is burned up at about one ounce an hour.

A three-pound chemical factory, the liver industriously metabolizes alcohol, manufactures proteins, acts as a storehouse for sugar, fats, and vitamins, filters the blood of impurities, and secretes bile into the intestines to aid digestion. The bewildering variety of its functions is still only dimly understood, although architectural maps of its crooked corridors and neatly dovetailed cells have

been available for hundreds of years. Trouble comes when globules of fat crowd the liver cells until they die. Scar tissue invades
and blocks the corridors, so that blood can no longer run freely,
and the manufacturing and storage centers are clogged into quies-
cence.

There are several ways this can happen. One is malnutrition.
Another is infection. The third is alcohol. It used to be thought
that malnutrition, not ethanol, caused the damage seen in many
alcoholics. They are notoriously careless eaters, and an impoverished diet is implicated in many cases of liver disease. But recent
research on baboons and men has clearly indicated that liquor can
make the chemical plant choke to a halt even when diet is adequate. Dr. Charles Lieber and his associates at the Mt. Sinai
School of Medicine in New York decided to try producing cirrhosis of the liver in laboratory animals. They had previously shown
that even well-nourished alcoholics developed fatty livers—easily
reversible and evidently not harmful. Now they wanted to go one
step further but, of course, could not subject human beings to the
dangers of irreversible damage. They decided to use baboons, who
have livers singularly similar to those of people. For four years
they plied their baboons (who lived in a trailer in the wooded hills
of New York's Sterling Forest) with both alcohol and a nutrition-
ally adequate diet. It took the full four years in some cases, but
some of the animals finally did develop cirrhosis, the first time an
animal experiment confirmed what many doctors had long sus-
pected. There are still skeptics who point out that even with a
good diet, the baboons (and the earlier male volunteers) could
have been undernourished, since alcohol keeps certain crucial factors such as vitamin B_{12}, folic acid, and magnesium from being
utilized by the body. Dr. Lieber is convinced it is the alcohol. This
kind of liver disease, which occurs almost exclusively in alcoholics,
is called Laënnec's cirrhosis, after the doctor in Napoleon's time
who first connected the scarring he found in autopsies with the illness he saw in living men. Considering the passionate French concern with the liver, it seems particularly fitting that a Frenchman's
name should identify the disease. (René Laënnec was not only an
astute observer, he is also famous for inventing the stethoscope.) A
man who drinks a pint of whiskey a day—the equivalent of four
or five stiff highballs—runs a fifty-fifty chance of developing

Laënnec's cirrhosis after twenty years, and the damage is irreversible.

When alcohol is metabolized by the liver, it first becomes acetaldehyde, a highly toxic substance that luckily is quickly transformed into acetate and then into what alcohol turns into in the outside world—acetic acid or vinegar. This is then transformed into harmless carbon dioxide and water. Antabuse, an antidrinking medication, works by blocking the switch from acetaldehyde, permitting that poison to build up and trigger consistently unpleasant, sometimes dangerous, side effects. The small amount of alcohol that is not burned up in the liver returns to the outside world unchanged as boozy breath, in sweat, and in urine. That's why breath tests are an accurate indicator of blood-alcohol levels.

As alcohol is oxidized by liver enzymes, hydrogen atoms are cast off. These are what mess up the cell chemistry of the body's largest organ, directly or indirectly, and start the drinker on her way to possible problems. Uric acid—associated with gout—builds up in the bloodstream, suggesting that sore-toe sufferers were right when they tied their attacks to tippling. More ominously, the excess hydrogen also encourages the production of fats. Faced with large amounts of both free hydrogen and fats, the liver opts for the free hydrogen, using it instead of the hydrogen in fats and allowing the fats to accumulate in its own cells and as cholesterol and triglycerides in the bloodstream. (Low doses of alcohol, however, may do just the reverse.) These globules have been implicated in heart disease. The fats in the liver itself seem harmless at first, but the baboon studies have shown that, if not interrupted, the crowding of liver cells by fat globules seems to promote alcoholic hepatitis (with cells dying) and finally, alcoholic cirrhosis.

But the remarkable liver is an accommodating organ. Early effects are reversible if the drinker just stops drinking for a few days. Without the interference of alcohol, it swiftly produces new cells to replace damaged ones, erasing all evidence of overindulgence.

One dangerous effect of drinking is really the result of liver damage, although it erupts in the throat. Since blood has a hard time coursing through blocked liver passageways, the other blood-carrying areas are overloaded. A common cause of death in cirrhosis is rupture of the veins in the esophagus.

Elsewhere in the gastrointestinal tract, an area of the body exquisitely susceptible to alcohol's effects, the results can be minor or life-threatening, depending, again, on the dosage. Hiccups, heartburn, vomiting, and stomach pains can hit the social drinker as well as the alcoholic. As Dr. Leon Greenberg of the Rutgers Center for Alcohol Studies emphasized, "Alcohol is an irritant, and every time someone takes a couple of martinis, he's whacking the inside of his stomach with a board."

On a hopeful note, there's no convincing evidence that alcohol causes ulcers, although it does, of course, irritate those that already exist.

Since so many of alcohol's bad effects have traditionally been blamed on malnutrition and since certain B vitamins are crucial in treating some effects, there have been attempts to treat alcoholism itself with vitamins. Some doctors have given megadoses with what they say is success. Nutritionist Carlton Fredericks suggests that since low blood sugar is present in alcoholics and, as he found, in some people before they become alcoholic, a diet to correct this aberration might end the alcoholism. These nutritional approaches have received neither controlled testing nor widespread acceptance.

High blood pressure is about 25 percent more prevalent among women than among men, and the first large-scale study of the relationship of drinking to this condition has now linked it to three or more drinks a day. More than eighty thousand men and women using the Kaiser-Permanente Medical Care Program in Oakland, California, answered routine health questionnaires that were then checked against their medical records and analyzed statistically. Men who had two or fewer drinks a day had blood pressure readings like those of abstainers. Women had even lower blood pressure than abstainers at this drinking rate. But once the intake reached three a day, both men and women had higher blood pressure. The findings do not prove a cause-and-effect relationship—the cause of most high blood pressure is still unknown. But the figures do demonstrate a connection of some sort. In a report in the *New England Journal of Medicine* (May 26, 1977), the epidemiologists concluded, "Our findings suggest that there may be a 'threshold level' of regular alcohol consumption (usual intake of three or more drinks per day in our categorization) above which blood-pressure elevations are found and below which pressures are not higher or perhaps slightly lower than in nondrinkers."

Complications from high blood pressure include strokes, blindness, kidney disease, and a heightened risk of heart attacks. The researchers don't comment directly on the intriguing finding that one or two drinks a day actually lowered women's blood pressure as the same alcohol dosage seems to lower the risk of heart attacks. White women who were better educated, smoked, or drank six or more cups of coffee a day also tended to have lower blood pressure—a paradox in the scientific world, where other studies implicate smoking and caffeine as harmful.

Attempts to induce cancer in animals by painting their skins with alcohol or exposing mice to 20 percent alcohol in their drinking water over a long period of time haven't worked. Alcohol itself does not seem to cause cancer directly, although it does increase the risk of the disease occurring in the mouth, throat, and stomach.[10] When its use is combined with smoking, the chance of developing cancer of the mouth or throat escalates a fearful fifteen times. Somehow the two substances act on each other in a way that makes the combined risk much greater than the two separate risks added together. The speculation is that alcohol is a catalyst, making it easier for some other carcinogen to cross the cell barrier. With alcohol alone, according to one study, the risk of cancer in these areas is six times greater from whiskey than from wine or beer. However, another study found that heavy drinkers who use only wine or beer have the highest risk. Dr. Julia Morton of the University of Miami found higher rates of stomach cancer in regular users of French red wines. Her guess is that it is the high tannin content that does the damage.

Paradoxically, alcohol is useful in diagnosing Hodgkin's disease, a cancer of the lymph tissues. Small doses can cause almost immediate pain at the site of the tumor. When the tumor is gone, so is the reaction to alcohol. A similar reaction has been found in another type of cancer. Dr. T. B. Brewin of the Glasgow, Scotland, Institute of Radiotherapeutics and Oncology found that sudden intolerance to alcohol—painful breathing, flushing, nausea, pain—could signal cancer of the cervix in certain cases, sometimes as much as two years before the diagnosis was made by more conventional methods. Women with cancer of the breast did not have this kind of reaction. Unfortunately, there has been no attempt to duplicate Dr. Brewin's study in this country, and Dr. John L. Lewis of the Memorial Sloan-Kettering Cancer Center in New

York is frankly skeptical of the results. Dr. Brewin counters with, "Nobody has denied it, but neither has anybody confirmed it. Apart from alcohol pain in Hodgkin's disease, which was the first thing to be described [by an American physician, who himself suffered from it], the subject lies dormant and more or less unrecognized. . . . There is certainly a lot more work to be done on the subject and a lot more to be discovered."

The same could be said of other areas. Is alcohol an aphrodisiac, for instance? Here, of course, it's important to separate attitudes from actions. Women who drink a lot are universally supposed to be sexually promiscuous. When she studied young women college students at Harvard, Dr. Sharon Wilsnack found that, true to barroom tradition, a few drinks made them feel more sexy and feminine. Stories made up on a psychological test administered to these women resembled the ones of nursing mothers—the ultimate in femininity. Other researchers found that in men, drinking triggered fantasies of power and strength, maybe because of the burning sensation of swallowing hard liquor plus the adrenalin released by the action of the drug. (Adrenalin is a hormone that has the capacity to charge the body up for a fight or to meet danger.) Put the sexually fantasizing women and the powerful men together and you get what everyone has always said you would get—an orgy, or at least seduction.

But do you? There is very little evidence to go on. As J. A. Carpenter and N. P. Armenti, two researchers who examined the sparse scientific literature on alcohol and sexual arousal, discovered, "Most experts comment on human sexual behavior and alcohol as though only males drink and have sexual interests." For the men, Shakespeare said it best when he wrote in *Macbeth*, "Lechery, sir, it provokes and unprovokes; it provokes the desire, but it takes away the performance." That a lot of alcohol leads to temporary impotence has been written into comedy routines ever since Macbeth's porter became such a hit. Now an ingenious experiment has shown that an equivalent effect may strike women.

Sixteen young women at Rutgers University in New Jersey volunteered to have their reaction to an erotic film and one that could have been rated "G" for general audiences monitored by G. Terence Wilson and David M. Lawton under gradually increasing doses of alcohol. Half of them were told that alcohol would cut down on their sexual arousal; the other half were told it would enhance it. They were all equipped with a tampon-sized vaginal photoplethysmograph to measure and record vaginal pulse and blood volume while they watched. The films had been specially selected to show women initiating the sexual action, with most of the emphasis on the woman—conditions other experimenters had found particularly exciting.

Inexorably, as the blood-alcohol level went up, vaginal indications of sexual arousal went down—just as they had in studies on men when a measure of penile tumescence was used. As a fascinating sidelight, the women who were told they would be more excited when intoxicated showed even fewer physical indications of arousal than those who were told the reverse. Like men, among whom more impotence has been reported by sex therapists since women began demanding equal satisfaction, the pressure to perform may have made it harder for these women to react. When they were given a battery of psychological tests to assess their sexual feelings, they repeated the results of the physical monitoring: As more alcohol was consumed, unconscious sexuality was dampened. But when they were simply asked about their feelings, more of them said they felt sexier with more alcohol—a clear indication that sexual satisfaction has more to do with what happens in the brain than in the body.

Probably these unromantic, objective tests results will have no effect at all on the hallowed use of alcohol as a sexual enhancer. In another study, a questionnaire without the control of physical measurements turned up these classic responses: 68 percent of the women reported that alcohol increased sexual pleasure; 11 percent said it had no effect; and 21 percent felt it decreased pleasure. Of the men (who may have been more dramatically aware of the physical effects of the drug), only 45 percent felt it was enhancing, 13 percent said it made no difference, and 42 percent saw it as lessening their enjoyment.[11]

Alcoholic women have always borne the brunt of the traditional association of drinking with promiscuity. But as Dr. Edith Gomberg, professor of social work at the University of Michigan, warns: "The issue of alcohol-and-sexual behavior is really two issues, one of knowledge, and one of attitudes. We do not actually know that women who become drunk or who are alcoholic are more likely to engage in sexual behavior. There are some pretty lurid case histories, but when physicians are asked about the sexual behavior of their alcoholic women patients they disagree among themselves, some reporting 'loose sexual morals' and others saying 'no.' Popular attitudes, however, are clearly negative; whatever the actual facts, attitudes toward women's drunkenness are negative and there is a strong popular belief that female drunkenness and loose sexual behavior are associated." [12]

This is true even among alcoholic men. As one counselor at a co-ed rehabilitation center put it, "The men see the women as tramps—the lowest of the low—certainly lower than they are, and fair game sexually." However, many alcoholic women report that, although they remain perpetually available, they are frigid, and Dr. Helen Singer Kaplan, one of this country's foremost sex therapists, has found that "habitual heavy intake frequently seriously impairs the sexual response in both genders."

Shakespeare's observation was evidently true for women as well as men: Alcohol may increase desire but interfere with satisfaction. If it is an aphrodisiac, it is a deceptive one. But myths about alcohol die hard. Despite the accumulation of scientific evidence, drinking is still supposed by many to save victims of exposure (a blanket would be better than the St. Bernard's cask of brandy), help fight the common cold (it disturbs the body's heat-regulating mechanism and may be harmful), and revive shock victims (in small doses it dangerously lowers blood pressure, making things worse). Hundreds of years of folklore stubbornly resist revision.

4

The Fight Against Demon Rum

*T*he drives for temperance and women's votes, joined in an
uneasy marriage, were the most successful political movements in American history. Within a year, constitutional
amendments providing for Prohibition (effective January 16, 1920)
and suffrage (effective August 20, 1920) were the law of the land.
The gentlemen, bless 'em, were of inestimable help, particularly
in the Anti-Saloon League. But the grassroots work was done by
women who fought against liquor and for the vote. Some of them
are now an embarrassment to those feminists who would rather
forget that almost every woman who led the march to the ballot
box got her training in the righteous halls of the temperance
movement.

As a college for teaching community organization, platform
speaking, and political lobbying, the temperance movement has
never been surpassed. And the moving force behind the fight
against Demon Rum was hardly the prim, sanctimonious church-
lady of the stereotypes. She was a militant radical who was not
afraid to speak out, to join black and white women together soon
after the Civil War, or to call—in a ladylike way, of course—for
woman to take her rightful place at the pinnacles of power.

She was tiny, just five feet three, with reddish hair pulled back
neatly into a knot. But she successfully led an army of virtuous,

white-ribboned women into the fight against alcohol, and then, almost to their own amazement, into the unpopular battle for women's rights and votes. Her name was Frances Willard, and her army called itself the Woman's Christian Temperance Union. She took over as president in 1879.

It wasn't the first temperance movement in this country, though. In 1808 Saratoga Springs, New York, reacted to Revolutionary War surgeon Benjamin Rush's pamphlet *Inquiry into the Effects of Ardent Spirits* with an organization to push for an end to the use of distilled liquor. Wine and beer were still too much a part both of life and the doctor's little black bag to come under attack. By 1836, though, the American Society for the Advancement of Temperance had come out against all alcoholic beverages, and the country was full of groups talking about and praying against the evils of drink. There were temperance societies of sailors and merchants. There was even a temperance group in Congress.[1]

But women carried the battle into the streets. They had a vested interest in the fight. Drinking was endemic among men in the nineteenth century, and men who drank spent all the family money, abused their wives and children, and often even made off with a wife's factory wages to spend in the saloon. On the frontier, a drunken husband meant an unprotected family, open to attack and even starvation. The teary, overblown barroom ballads were only slight exaggerations of the painful truth. Women with drunken husbands were helpless. In most states they had no property rights, not even over money they earned themselves; divorce was a disgrace and couldn't be requested by the woman; and children could not be taken from their fathers. Wives were utterly dependent—as dependent, one orator pointed out, as the black slaves had been. It's not surprising then that in the 1870s women were still dependent on a man to mobilize their anger and despair.

Dr. Dioclesian Lewis inspired the woman's crusade at a temperance lecture in Hillsboro, New York. A Harvard graduate, inventor of the beanbag, and a handsome, white-haired inveigher against the evils of drink, he roused his audience with the story of how his sainted mother and some of her friends had fallen to their knees in front of a local saloon and shamed the owner into closing his doors. In fifty days, praying women closed 150 saloons in upstate New York and Ohio. Of course, the saloons reopened almost as quickly as the bonnets and bustles disappeared from the doorways, but the movement had begun. The people who laughed at the sentimental songs and maudlin appeals were soon in awe of the power of righteous women on the march.

At a meeting on the serene shores of New York's Lake Chatauqua (temperance always was more a rural than a big-city movement, and upstate New York, for some strange reason, its cradle), the ladies of the National Sunday School Association decided to form what finally became the Woman's Christian Temperance Union (WCTU). That same year, in 1874, Frances Willard fell to her knees in the sawdust of a saloon in Pittsburgh, Pennsylvania, and intoned her first public prayer. Temperance was a part of her heritage; as a child she had signed this vow, inscribed in the family Bible:

> *A pledge we make, no wine to take,*
> *Nor brandy red that turns the head,*
> *Nor fiery rum that ruins home,*
> *Nor whiskey hot that makes the sot,*
> *Nor brewers beer, for that we fear,*
> *And cider, too, will never do;*
> *To quench our thirst we'll always bring*
> *Cold water from the well or spring.*
> *So here we pledge perpetual hate*
> *To all that can intoxicate.*[2]

This temperate tomboy, who had hunted with her older brother as a pioneer's daughter, was involved early in unpopular causes. She had carried out progressive ideas as dean of the Woman's College of Northwestern University, but was finally forced out when her authority was threatened by the university's president, once her fiancé (she never married). She refused to be the first president of the WCTU, preferring to act as corresponding secretary and to build her power base. When she did take over the organization, she led, goaded, and pushed it until her death nineteen years later.

In a summary of recent sociological studies, one expert pointed out that if a woman wants to be a success, she should be a tomboy at some point in her life. She could have been talking about Frances Willard, whose *How to Win: A Book for Girls* exhorted them to assert their autonomy. She was a rousing speaker who added musical flourishes and flowers to dramatize what might have been humdrum meetings. Women, locked in domesticity, flocked to march behind her because she was exciting—and, of course, she was right.

Miss Willard's motto was "Do Everything." The WCTU not only fought the liquor traffic and worked for the vote; it established kindergartens and day-care centers; set up the first temperance hospital in this country based on the treatment of disease without alcohol, which was then considered medically indispensable; campaigned for and got (in Portland, Maine) the first police matrons; paid for matrons in Chicago until the city could afford the expense; and then suggested that women be allowed to walk a beat.

Frozen orange juice, strategically located drinking fountains, and McDonald's hamburgers also owe their existence, in one way or another, to the temperance movement. The ladies of the WCTU are credited with the fruit-juice industry because they campaigned against wine at communion, suggesting grape juice instead; drinking fountains with three levels—for birds, people, and dogs—cut down on beer as a thirst quencher; and when they went after the saloon, they also wiped out the free lunch—the hard-boiled eggs and pickled pigs' feet that used to grace the noontime counter. The result? The quick-lunch place where a man could get a sandwich and coffee instead of a schooner of beer and the trimmings. Even the All-American soda fountain was an attempt to compete with the bar.

All their fervor was directed at women as victims of alcohol, not users. The only hint that women, too, might be alcoholic came in the drive for police matrons to take care of those women who had fallen into the gutter. Even these were seen as victimized by a man, though. This attitude was immortalized in a famous series of Temperance engravings showing the decline and fall of the Latimer family. A happy, middle-class husband, wife, and children sank lower and lower as alcohol worked its Evil. The husband lost his job, the youngest child died of neglect, and finally Mrs. Latimer herself succumbed to drink and died as the result of a fight with her drunken husband. He ended his life "a hopeless maniac."

The WCTUers were, in a way, correct. Alcohol was largely a problem for women who were tied to alcoholic men. In the nineteenth century, opium, not strong drink, was the drug of choice for a woman, and there were more female opium addicts than male ones. Like playwright Eugene O'Neill's mother, women were innocently addicted by doctors who prescribed the then-legal drug for "female complaints." Like Mrs. O'Neill, too, they tried to keep their men from drowning in drink. They never touched a drop themselves (except whatever was hidden in patent remedies). And they crusaded against it.

Women joined the temperance movement for many reasons. Some of them, like Frances Willard, came out of a Puritan background that condemned drinking. Some were fighting foreign hordes—new European immigrants who brought beer-drinking and saloons with them. Others had drunken husbands or brothers or fathers or had seen neighborhood families destroyed. Still others, like WCTU leader Matilda B. Carse of Chicago, joined to fight the alcohol business. Her three-year-old son was killed when he was run over by a brewery wagon.

In 1876 the movement got a big boost when Rutherford B. Hayes was elected to the White House by the smallest possible margin—one electoral vote. Undaunted by this meager mandate, his WCTU wife, "Lemonade Lucy," determined to set an example of sobriety for the country. The first thing she did was to have the sideboard put down in the cellar; there was to be no strong drink stored in her house. Then she prohibited alcohol, even at formal dinners. For White House regulars and visiting diplomats this was a hardship comparable to being assigned to a mission in Siberia, but they were helped out in secret by a White House steward whose job it was to prepare the ices that cleansed the palate. Along with the lemon juice, he slipped in a generous quantity of rum. The regulars called this pause that refreshed "The Lifesaving Station."

There were many homes around the country that were as dry as the White House seemed to be. They, and their families, signed the official WCTU pledge: "I hereby solemnly promise, God helping me, to abstain from all distilled, fermented, and malt liquors, including wine, beer, and cider, and to employ all proper means to discourage the use of and traffic in the same." Temperance roused the respectable women of the country to action, particularly in small towns and rural areas, and if men drank they had to do it outside the home and face having their names written down if they went into the local saloon. In Ohio, the women of one temperance society supplemented the standard pledge with one that was usually shortened to "Lips that touch liquor shall never touch mine"—enough to discourage any suitor tempted by strong drink.

When women got into temperance, it changed. Instead of the movement advocating moderation in drinking (as it had when men were in charge) it came down hard on the side of total abstinence. There was no middle way. Alcohol was a poison that rotted the brain, paralyzed the will, and destroyed the family. It was unique, evil, and endemic. It had to be wiped out. Along with this stiff-necked moral outrage went a picture of the user of this awful stuff. The drinker had fallen from grace into the gutter, had committed a terrible sin, and must ask forgiveness. Despite more modern psychological and scientific understanding, the legacy of these old standards and attitudes still colors today's picture of the person who drinks too much.

The moral outrage generated in the fight against alcohol was harnessed by Frances Willard for another cause; she dragged the conservative WCTU, kicking and screaming a little, into the not quite respectable fight for women's suffrage. She began quietly enough. In 1881 she suggested that women should have the right to vote—but only on temperance issues—so they could protect home and family against the evils of the saloon. Susan B. Anthony had early suggested at a temperance convention that "The way to handle these problems was to give women the right to divorce alcoholic husbands, the right to keep their own earnings, and, above all, the right to vote for these rights which men would not, of their own volition, give to women." [3] At the 1888 International Council of Women, on a platform that she shared with Mrs. Anthony, Frances Willard issued her own ringing call to action: "I believe that whatever may come out of this mighty conflict [between wets and drys] in which women and temperance are so largely synonymous, there is to come 'no sex in citizenship.' I believe that we are to find that since the ballot is the emblem of power, since majorities must decide what the law shall be, we want woman as a voter and law-maker."

It is a peculiarly American paradox that most of the early fighters for women's emancipation began as soldiers in the battle against Demon Rum. Susan B. Anthony soon focused her energies on votes; Frances Willard continued to be firmly and publicly committed to both Prohibition and suffrage. Ironically, the movement of women into wider participation in politics led them also into wider participation in drinking, hardly what the WCTU had in mind.

This partnership of temperance and women's rights led to unexpected consequences. The brewers and distillers decided that votes for women would inevitably mean Prohibition, and they launched and financed an attack that undoubtedly delayed women's suffrage. To raise money, they added special taxes on their barrels of beer and whiskey; with per capita consumption at more than two gallons of whiskey and seventeen of beer a year, this provided a substantial reservoir of funds to fight those twin evils, votes for women and Prohibition. They used other methods, too. In some states saloon keepers had to kick in to provide campaign funds against the ladies. There were also threats, blackmail, and boycotts in the fight to save the free-enterprise system, male supremacy, and the sanctity of the saloon. The ladies, meanwhile, kept pointing out, as Frances Willard did shortly before her death, "We must have a national prohibitory amendment, so that we can ground our principles in the organic law of the highest legislature of our land, thus making the liquor traffic an Esau, an Ishmaelite and a social Pariah in this land." One militant prohibitionist went after the evil alcohol industry by saying, "Women believe in prevention rather than cure and they are not willing to be the mop of the liquor traffic. We are sympathetic and willing to help any drunkard. But we think it better to turn off the spigot than to mop up the floor."

Carry Nation's thesis was that it was best to start by smashing the spigot. This religious fanatic charged into the battle, eleven years after Frances Willard's death, as one anointed by God and given the job of destroying the rum traffic in the United States. Mrs. Nation's first husband had died of alcoholism. And she had seen visions (nothing particularly unusual in a family with a mother convinced she was Queen Victoria) instructing her to fight the devil. On June 6, 1900, as a member in good standing of her local WCTU chapter in Medicine Lodge, Kansas, she gathered up bricks and rocks she had wrapped in newspapers, added four heavy bottles to her ammunition, and drove into nearby Kiowa in her buggy to start her mission. For openers she smashed out the windows of three saloons, declaring they were in violation of the law (Kansas was dry) and therefore could not have the law's protection.

During her nine-year career as an avenging angel, she was arrested twenty-five times by her own reckoning for breaking and entering. With the hatchet with which she chopped open kegs of brandy and beer and her battle cry of "Smash, women, for the love of Jesus, smash," she became the rallying point for hundreds who followed her brawny six-foot figure into the saloons. As they marched they sang:

> *I stand for prohibition,*
> *The utter demolition*
> *Of all this curse of misery and woe;*
> *Complete extermination,*
> *Entire annihilation—*
> *The saloon must go!*

To help the saloon on its way to hell, grim-faced Carry traveled around the country, smashing, lecturing, and selling monogrammed pewter replicas of her famous weapon. Like the radicals of the 1960s she took the law into her own hands to call attention to evil, and undoubtedly helped polarize public opinion against strong drink.

When she went to Yale to investigate a shocking report that the students were being served sauces containing wine, she was photographed with some of the boys, glass in hand. Doctored to make it look as if Carry were about to down a stein of beer, this picture now hangs over the bar at New York's Yale Club, a reminder of how what began as a holy crusade turned into a craze, then into a circus, good for laughs. But, as the inscription on the gravestone of this woman who died insane in 1911 reads, "She Hath Done What She Could." Probably she had done a great deal. When Prohibition snuck up on the country in 1920, Carry's contribution to its almost universal lip-service popularity was finally recognized. She had made the fight against liquor vivid and memorable and had shown that women could do more than pray to get what they wanted. Her prowess was recorded in a poem by one of her admirers, Dr. T. J. Merryman:

When those who should enforce the law,
Are useless as are men of straw,
What force can make saloons withdraw?
A woman.

Women power had helped bring about the dual victories of votes and Prohibition, and it seemed that the forces of good had finally triumphed over the forces of evil. Organized against alcohol as the destroyer of family life, women had won themselves the right to be heard politically about this and any other issue they felt was important. It was a mythical victory, built on a supreme irony. The fight against alcohol hadn't defeated drink; it had, unexpectedly, brought women out of the parlor and into the streets to take their places next to men, feet on the rail, elbows on the bar. The fight for the vote, instead of bringing women to political power, just gave them one more area in which to reflect their husbands' thinking. What happened in the 1920s (a decade newspaperman Henry Lee called "the longest, saddest, wettest, craziest, funniest, bloodiest adventure in reform in American history") was that many women now thought delinquency was delightful. Defiance of the law they had so recently supported left behind a permanent distaste for legislating morality. Prohibition was probably the most widely flouted federal legislation in this country's history.

The final push toward the impossible goal of regulating people to perfection began quietly enough. World War I with its anti-German (anti-beer) feeling; the need for grain as food, not drink; and the reality that a sober soldier lives longer, all had helped the cause. But once the Prohibition Proclamation had been signed and the silver pen given to Anna A. Gordon, president of the WCTU, in recognition of women's role, the stage was set for scuttling the Great Experiment. Almost everyone had assumed that liquor would disappear from the American scene; instead, defiance of the law became a way of life, causing a revolution in mores and the phenomenal growth of a new industry—organized crime. New York's police commissioner estimated that in 1929, almost a decade after the start of Prohibition, the city had 32,000 speakeasies—about twice as many places to drink in as in the old days of the legal saloon. The owners got their supplies from rum runners who got them from the ships sitting off Long Island loaded with illicit liquor.

There was a vast network for making, shipping, protecting, and collecting on this illegal traffic, and the gangsters soon muscled in on the profits. They were considerable. One estimate was that, based on "government statistics and a personal survey," people were drinking more than ever before. In *Collier's Weekly*, a leading magazine, writer J. O'Donnell said that Americans consumed thirty million more gallons of alcoholic beverages in 1923 than in 1917, the last year of unrestricted production. And just before the saloons were padlocked the liquor industry (including beer production) had been the fifth largest in the country, grossing close to a billion dollars a year.

Of course, the drys kept insisting that post-Prohibition consumption figures were inflated and pointed out (probably accurately) that drunkenness had decreased among the working classes. In New York City, the number of women drunks arrested in 1918 was 1,495. During Prohibition it never again came near that peak. There is no question that deaths from cirrhosis of the liver (the standard disease of drinkers) also decreased.

Dr. Donald Goodwin, a psychiatrist who specializes in research on alcoholism, is on the side of the drys when he says this precipitous drop showed that, "In some ways, it [Prohibition] was a huge success." What seems to have happened is that the areas of the country that were wet became wetter; those that were dry before Prohibition stayed dry or became dryer. Law-abiding, God-fearing citizens gave up their occasional cocktail but the young and fashionable discovered that alcohol mixed well with Freudian psychology, the movies, and the roadster. Despite the fact that accurate statistics are not available, there seems little doubt that in certain groups, at least, drinking increased. The most revolutionary change came among women.

Before the country went dry, drinking (except for a little sherry or port) was unusual for women, and the local bar or saloon was strictly a male hangout. A woman who walked into one was assumed (usually correctly) to be a prostitute looking for business.

With Prohibition, a lot of this changed. Drinking became the thing to do in certain groups—a little naughty, but nice. Breaking the law wasn't hard, it was fun. And, for the first time, men and women began sharing the fun of having a few drinks in public together. Elmer Davis, later an outstanding radio commentator, wrote at this time, "The old days when father spent his evenings at

Cassidy's bar with the rest of the boys are gone, and probably gone forever; Cassidy may still be in business at the old stand, and father may still go down there of evenings, but since Prohibition mother goes with him."

It wasn't only Cassidy's bar that flourished. Manufacturers of hip flasks that could be carried conveniently to football games and on automobile rides (another contributor to the change in social values) found their products in demand. Women's dresses were designed with pockets so they could carry their own supplies, and John Held, Jr., clever chronicler of the Age of the Flapper, captioned one of his line drawings "the flapper who is willing to try any pocket flask once." Speakeasies flourished behind grilled doors whose slots slid open to admit only friendly faces. With Scotch and rye selling at six, seven, or eight dollars a bottle, gin soon soared in popularity. It cost only twenty dollars a dozen.

People who had drunk only at home now came out and joined in the general hilarity in the relaxed, "let's all have fun" atmosphere of the illegal drinking place. Women were customers, owners, and entertainers. Probably the most famous of them all was Mary Louise Cecilia Guinan, the tall blond beauty from Texas who greeted her patrons with a drawled, "Hello, sucker." Her New York place—shifting from building to building as one spot after another was padlocked by federal agents—offered pretty girls, entertainment ("Now I wantcha to give this little girl a great big hand"), and liquor for all. At least, that's what the Prohibition agents said. Texas Guinan maintained until her death that she never sold alcohol in her clubs and that she never drank it, either.

Most women didn't drink, but for many of those who did, the drink had shifted from genteel sherry to gin or cocktails of one kind or another. They drank with men and found that a little alcohol made the whole world seem friendlier. To poke fun at the tireless members of the WCTU and Anti-Saloon League, men and women raised their glasses and flasks in speakeasies and living rooms and sang this classic:

> *We're coming, we're coming, our brave little band;*
> *On the right side of temp'rance we now take our stand.*
> *We don't use tobacco because we all think,*
> *That the people who do so are likely to drink!*
> *[They were right]* . . .

We never eat fruitcake because it has rum.
And one little slice puts a man on the bum.
Oh can you imagine a sorrier sight
Than a man eating fruitcake until he gets tight?*

The noble effort to end the evil trade in rum was obviously a resounding failure. One vaudevillian quipped, "Sure I'm in favor of Prohibition. I wish they'd try it sometime."

There was still a lot of dry sentiment around, and most people assumed that women, as defenders of the family, would try to hang onto Prohibition until by some miracle it was effective. But there were also women on the other side of the question who saw what a farce the federal regulations were and who worked for legalization of liquor. They were led by socialite Mrs. Charles H. Sabin, first woman member of the Republican National Committee, who resigned her post to campaign for a return to sanity. She got almost a million and a half—the Sabin Women—to follow her, and with their help the country went wet again on December 5, 1933.

What Prohibition had done for women was break down a few of the barriers that had kept them from being the full, equal drinking partners of men. But despite co-ed drinking and passing out in speakeasies and on the back seats of cars, the equality was more apparent than real. Women who drank were considered smart or modern, particularly in the big cities, but they were also looked at critically. (In Muncie, Indiana, America's Middletown, sociologist Robert Lynd found in 1933 that "smoking and drinking are more appropriate leisure-time activities for men than for women.") Women who drank too much were—and still are—seen as morally and emotionally weak. Still, it was only after Prohibition that the WCTU—and others—recognized the possibility that alcohol consumption might cause problems for women other than those who were on skid row.

But despite today's lip service to the idea that alcoholism is a disease and not a defect of the will, the attitudes of what Selden D. Bacon of Rutgers University named "the Classic Temperance movement" are still with us. Even doctors, supposedly aware and nonjudgmental, tend to ignore or not look for signs of alcohol abuse in middle-class patients. "Nice" people don't have problems with drinking. It is a skid-row phenomenon and a moral defect, as the WCTU kept pointing out. This legacy has continued to set the tone for American ambivalence about alcohol and, as Dr. Bacon emphasizes, had its "greatest impact . . . perhaps upon the users of alcohol. They too accepted the Movement's message." Particularly for women, the message has been: "You are bad. You should feel guilty." This had been reinforced by society. As actress Mercedes McCambridge (a recovered alcoholic) recalled, she was seen as "some kind of moral leper, some kind of spiritual wreck, a rather unattractive blot casting a dark shadow on the glistening perfection that is the rest of society. . . ."

5

Who Becomes Alcoholic?

*M*ore women are drinking than ever before. But are they drinking more and having more problems? Probably. There are estimates that the number of women alcoholics compared to the number of men alcoholics has soared from a proportion of one woman to five men to one woman to three men, and even, according to some observers, one to one. Alcoholics Anonymous reports that in 1974, 33 percent of its new members were women, and in some urban areas, this figure reached the uncomfortable parity of 50 percent. In other parts of the world, too, the numbers are rising; in Australia one treatment agency says its case load has tripled in the last five years. It's impossible to tell whether this means that there are more women alcoholics or only that they are now freer to come out of the kitchen. Dr. Sharon Wilsnack comes down on the side of greater visibility. After completing a national study on women and drinking in 1981, she commented emphatically, "There is no evidence over the past decade of a dramatic increase or 'epidemic' of heavy drinking or drinking problems among women." The one potentially ominous trend she did find was a significantly higher percentage of women aged thirty-five to forty-nine who were heavier drinkers. If this persists it would be a sign of increased problems with alcohol in middle-aged

women.[1] Of the estimated 14 million alcoholics and problem
drinkers in this country, more than 3.5 million are said to be
women. The number of still-hidden drinking women is, of course,
unknown, but in wealthy, suburban Fairfield County, Connecti-
cut, the guess is there are nine at home for every one who asks for
help.

There's also the possibility that a growing bureaucracy (the National Institute on Alcohol Abuse and Alcoholism was founded in
1970) has an investment in keeping the problem before the public.
Growing awareness may not necessarily mean a growing problem.
As one academic expert commented wryly, "Women are good politics." Jan DuPlain, first head of the National Council on Alcoholism (NCA) office on women, however, estimated that 50 percent of
the reported increase is due to awareness, the other half to a real
increase in the number of women alcoholics.

A major problem with all these estimates is the disagreement as
to what constitutes alcoholism. As Humpty-Dumpty said to Alice
in Wonderland (and many researchers seem to repeat it when pre-
senting their conclusions), "When I use a word, it means just what
I choose it to mean—neither more nor less." It is, therefore, almost
impossible to count "alcoholics" or to say there are more or fewer
than there were some years ago if there is no clear understanding
of who should be counted.

The question isn't simply one of semantics; it goes to the heart
of the matter. Is alcoholism a disease? If it is a disease, what are its
symptoms and outcome? Should it be treated only by physicians?
If it is a complex condition involving an interaction among personal problems, genetics, social attitudes, and cultural conditioning, who is most likely to succumb to these influences? What
distinguishes this condition from heavy social drinking? What direction should research take? Who gets the money? And finally,
depending on the definition of what alcoholism really is, how can
it best be prevented and, if not prevented, treated?

Everybody in Nancy's social group does a lot of drinking. There
are one or two drinks before lunch, cocktails before dinner, wine, a
nightcap. Weekends are party times. She's never missed a day of
work, but she's never missed a day of drinking, either.

Is this alcoholism?

*   *   *

Cathy hides the empties, then takes them in the trunk of her car to the recycling center. The children get themselves off to school in the morning and expect her to sleep until they get home. Her husband has stopped taking her to business parties because her behavior is unpredictable.

Is this alcoholism?

There are months when Millie doesn't drink at all. Then there are the times she doesn't remember much about. She had two glasses of champagne at her daughter's wedding and kept drinking until she had to be put to bed.

Is this alcoholism?

It all depends. Although the stereotyped alcoholic who cannot get along without the drug—the alcohol addict—is universally recognized, the questions involve people who are not at that point on the scale. The World Health Organization defines alcoholics as "those excessive drinkers whose dependence upon alcohol has attained such a degree that it shows a noticeable mental disturbance or an interference with their bodily and mental health, their interpersonal relations, and their smooth social and economic functioning; or who show the prodromal [warning] signs of such development." This wide-ranging net has been criticized as being so vague it cannot be useful in winnowing out who is and who is not a victim of what the WHO (along with the American Medical Association) accepts as a disease which, if untreated, progresses inexorably to premature death. Untreated male alcoholics, it is generally agreed, cut their lives short by ten to twelve years and women cut theirs by about fifteen years.

Mrs. Marty Mann, founder of the National Council on Alcoholism, the first citizens' group to deal with this problem, said, "An alcoholic is someone whose drinking causes a continuing problem in any department of his or her life." The key word here, she pointed out, is *continuing*. She added that alcoholism is a disease that, like diabetes, can be controlled but not cured. In her view, there are people who may seem to be alcoholics but really are not. They include the situational drinker who drinks heavily after a family tragedy she finds impossible to bear and then stops once she has regained her psychic balance, and the mentally ill for whom heavy drinking is a kind of self-medication that masks other symptoms.

More succinctly, psychiatrist J. A. Smith says, "In essence, any individual who relies on alcohol to meet the ordinary demands of living and continues to drink after alcohol has caused [her] marital or occupational difficulty is an alcoholic, whether [she] drinks only in the evening, has never taken a drink when alone, or has not touched anything but beer for five years."

Alcoholism as a disease, then, is identified by its social consequences as well as by the damage it may do to physical systems. This way of looking at it was formulated in the 1940s by Yale physiologist E. M. Jellinek, who first outlined the disorder in a systematic way, listed the symptom clusters through which it progresses, and gave the disease concept an official base.

According to Jellinek, there are four types of alcoholism: The Alpha type is represented by those who use alcohol continuously for emotional reasons. Alphas do not lose control of their drinking, although they may drink more than others in their social group. The Beta type is distinguished by physical symptoms: cirrhosis of the liver, stomach upsets. But the person need not be addicted and may show no withdrawal symptoms. Gamma alcoholism is the type generally accepted by Alcoholics Anonymous as the real thing. There are "craving," loss of control over drinking, and withdrawal symptoms if drinking stops. One psychologist who treats alcoholics says of this type of person, "She can't help drinking any more than someone with a cold can help sneezing." Probably, Jellinek says, Gamma is the predominant type in the United States and Canada. Delta alcoholism is much like Gamma, except that the drinker does not necessarily drink herself into death or oblivion, but has to maintain a certain level of alcohol intake and can't abstain.

Through the years, Jellinek's formulations have been modified and, in some cases, narrowed. The definition of alcoholism as a disease has usually been reserved for the "loss of control" type. Long before Jellinek, the classic sufferer from this condition was vividly described in the Book of Proverbs (13:29–35):

Who hath woe? Who hath sorrow? Who hath contentions? Who hath babbling? Who hath wounds without cause?

[Today, unexplained bruises in women are one sign of the hidden alcoholic.] Who hath redness of eyes?

"They that tarry along at the wine; they that go to seek mixed wine. . . . At the last it biteth like a serpent, and stingeth like an adder. . . . They have stricken me, thou shalt say, and I was not sick; they have beaten me, and I felt it not; when shall I awake? I will seek it yet again."

In arguing for the view that alcoholism of the kind the Bible described is itself a disease and not just a symptom of another malady, Mark Keller, an associate of Jellinek and for many years editor of the *Quarterly Journal of Studies on Alcohol,* replied to critics with this indignant rebuttal:

But is alcoholism a disease? I think it is (and well named alcoholism, and I wouldn't attach the label alcoholism to anything that isn't a disease). I think it is a disease because the alcoholic can't consistently choose whether or not he shall engage in a self-injurious behavior—that is, any of the alcoholismic drinking patterns. I think of it as a psychological disablement. And I don't think physical dependence or tolerance or altered cell metabolism (in which I can't believe on the basis of the evidence up to now) have anything to do with the case. . . . Nor does it bother me that there are stages in alcoholism, or a variety of developmental courses, or various degrees of severity, or different orders and combinations of manifestations, or that the symptoms (including loss of control) don't operate twenty-four hours a day 365 days a year. There are lots of diseases with such inconstant characteristics, and not only psychological diseases—for example, tuberculosis and diabetes.

Despite this eloquence, researchers who need clear criteria for deciding who is and who isn't alcoholic within the population they want to study are not quite convinced. Sociologist Kaye Fillmore says, "One of the real problems in this field is that no one can say Mrs. Jones or Miss Smith is an alcoholic until she says so herself or is having withdrawal symptoms."

Unlike researchers, the general public is not willing to wait that long, or to get mired in the experts' arguments about how much drinking, or how much loss of control, or how many lost jobs, constitute alcoholism—or whether it is a disease, a symptom of some other psychological disorder, or a bad habit. Having looked at the differing viewpoints there is now nothing to do but pretend they don't exist and plod along with the standard words—*disease* and *alcoholism.* Otherwise the little that is known about this condition gets lost in controversy.

Emerging through all the verbiage is this simple reality: An alcoholic is someone whose life is controlled by alcohol. She is not in charge, the drug is. And there is one other reality on which most treatment approaches are based: Without alcohol, there can be no alcoholism. Abstinence is the surest way out of the destructive cycle. Regular customers at a working-class tavern in the Midwest, whose attitudes were studied for five years by sociologist E. E. Masters, have these clear-cut criteria for determining what kind of behavior distinguishes the alcoholic woman from the social drinker: Does the woman neglect her children as a result of excessive drinking? Does she become sexually promiscuous when drinking? (The shadow of the pedestal again.)

Despite today's reevaluation of the disease concept, there is agreement that it has been useful in removing some of the "fallen woman" stigma surrounding alcoholism. Some general hospitals now accept alcoholic patients, and insurance companies pay for treatment. By the late 1970s public drunkenness was no longer a crime in thirty-six states, and scientific research on alcohol and women is respectable. For alcoholics themselves the understanding that what they are struggling with is closer to diabetes than to sin can help lift the load of guilt.

Underneath the surface acceptance of the medical model, however, the old moralistic attitudes about "lack of willpower" and "moral weakness" persist. Actress Mercedes McCambridge recalled that when her family learned she was an alcoholic, they saw her disease as "shameful, it is dirty and I am a dirty word." Almost all the studies agree that women alcoholics are seen as "worse" than men and greeted with greater condemnation. For both men and women there is still the legacy of the "all you have to do is stop" attitude, which assumes the alcoholic is lazy or deficient in willpower or has no pride. A man Dr. Vernon Johnson treated related that his wife "thought I could [stop drinking] if I would but that I wouldn't, and I knew that I would if I could, but I couldn't."

In an attempt to remove even more of the stigma, there has been a growing movement to modify the disease concept in favor of additional ways of looking at the condition. Mark Keller, defender of the traditional view, has dismissed these as part of the antimedical, antipsychiatric climate of the 1970s, but Don Cahalan, the sociologist who has done the only nationwide study of American drinking practices, points out that "alcoholics labeled as such under the disease concept are still considered poor risks as patients by many in the medical fraternity; thus it appears that the disease approach to alcohol problems has not as yet made material inroads on solving the problems. Hence many in the medical profession, as well as others in public health and the other healing arts, readily concede that a new or supplementary approach to drinking problems is in order." [2]

Despite more than thirty years of vigorous advocacy, the disease concept has not been able to erase the old attitudes about alcoholism and, according to some critics, may even have multiplied some of the alcoholic's problems. Fewer than half the doctors in private practice with an interest in alcoholism characterized it as a disease in a recent survey. After a look at a number of studies that chart the natural history of drinking patterns, Drs. K. W. Wanberg, J. L. Horn, and F. M. Foster of the University of Denver concluded that "a concept of alcoholism which assumes that there is a progressive illness is an oversimplification of a complex process. Acceptance of this concept can lead to an incorrect belief that there is only one best cure." And, they point out, although constant heavy drinking may lead to addiction, this isn't necessarily so. Winston Churchill, of course, is the favorite example of those who are struck by the fact that there are people who can drink large quantities every day and not suffer the usual dire consequences—physically, mentally, or socially. Some experts feel that people in need of help may have avoided it because they believed the orthodox view of "once an alcoholic, always an alcoholic." One psychiatrist uses the term "problem drinker" because, he says, "A diagnosis of alcoholism is worse than a diagnosis of cancer for some people." As a matter of fact, there is evidence that early death is not necessarily inevitable. And some experts question the policy of telling all alcoholics that even one drink leads inevitably to loss of control—especially when the belief has little basis in fact. (These studies on loss of control are discussed in chapter 10.)

If alcoholism is not necessarily characterized by loss of control or inevitable progression, and may or may not be a disease, what alternative ways are there of looking at it?

Since no one begins to drink heavily at birth, drinking must be something people learn. And, say the followers of the psychologist B. F. Skinner, what is learned can be unlearned if the rewards are immediate and pleasant enough. They can also be unlearned if the rewards are immediate and unpleasant enough. To the adherents of this school of thought, alcoholism is a bad habit, like nail-biting or compulsive talking, and can be corrected with the help of techniques developed in behavior modification or behavior therapy. In opposition to this view is that of Dr. Vernon Johnson, whose book *I'll Quit Tomorrow* has become a classic description of alcoholics and their treatment. Dr. Johnson says many women have told him, " 'I tried to keep up with my husband's drinking, but I couldn't do it. I threw up all over the living room.' So many people who try to become alcoholic fail. It just isn't something you learn from someone else."

Another way of looking at alcoholism comes out of systems theory—the psychological school which sees emotional problems as emerging out of a disordered "system"—the family, for instance. It used to be assumed that the wife or husband of the married alcoholic was either a victim or the cause of the alcoholism. Now there is research that indicates this just isn't so: *Both* have something to gain by holding on to the problem. In Dr. Murray Bowen's view, then, the whole system (the whole family) must be examined and treated before the alcoholic can change his or her behavior.

The lack of clarity and agreement about just what can be categorized as alcoholism, and whether it is a physical or psychological disease, a symptom of another underlying disease process, socially determined—or what have you—has had effects on attitudes, treatment, and even research. To sidestep these obstacles, sociologist Don Cahalan has also proposed scrapping the term "alcoholism" altogether and substituting "problem drinking." This would eliminate the loaded "sick" label and provide an opportunity to explore all the possible causes and consequences of the condition. He has developed a checklist of specific behavior patterns. If seven or more of them appear at the same time in the life of the same person, he would classify that person as a problem drinker.

First is frequent intoxication. Second, binge drinking, which he defines as being drunk for more than one day at a time. (Some studies show that women are more likely than men to have this drinking pattern.) Third, symptomatic drinking behavior, which includes physical dependence and loss of control. Fourth, physical dependence, or using alcohol habitually to handle the depression, nervousness, or stresses of daily living. Fifth, problems with spouse or relatives because of drinking. Sixth, the same kind of trouble with friends or neighbors. Seventh, trouble centering on work or unemployment. Eighth, problems with the police (while driving, on the job, at home) after someone is hurt. Ninth, health problems that have led a doctor to say "Cut down or you'll be in real trouble." Tenth, financial problems. Eleventh, belligerence or fighting. No one knows how many of these areas really apply to women (since most of what is known about drinking is based on men) but on the basis of these trouble spots, Cahalan found that 15 percent of men and 4 percent of women had clusters of seven or more problems. This would place the ratio of problem-drinking men to problem-drinking women at about 3.7 to 1. Others estimate that 2 to 3.5 million American women abuse alcohol.

Are Cahalan's "problem drinkers" alcoholic by the old standard? Is there a thin line that separates the social drinker from the alcoholic, or is it a chasm? Here again, it's a matter of choosing your expert. Dr. Morris Chafetz, former director of the NIAAA in Washington, says in *Why Drinking Can Be Good for You*, "Some say that only a hairline separates the social or moderate drinker from the alcoholic. Don't you believe it—a Grand Canyon separates them. . . . Drinking does not take the edge off reality just for the alcoholic; it does so for everyone or no one would do it." The crucial difference, he says, is in their definitions of reality. One sees it as a dull grind that can use a little brightening, the other finds it an unbearable burden. "One thing is certain," he adds, "the social drinker is in the vast majority."

Marty Mann, herself a former alcoholic, saw a chasm, too. The difference for her was that the social drinker (even one whose drinking is heavy) stays at pretty much the same level of consumption year after year. The alcoholic's pattern changes, progressing to disaster. Dr. Donald L. Gerard sees another distinguishing factor. The alcoholic says he drinks to be convivial, to relax, to put the tensions of the day behind him. He says he doesn't want to become drunk. But instead of achieving the universally desired glow, he becomes "unkempt, slovenly, stuporous and so on." The discrepancy between what he says he wants and what he achieves is enormous.

On the other hand, recent studies of large groups of drinkers— not necessarily alcoholic—have indicated that problem drinking (or alcoholism) is part of a continuum. It develops with time and, in some cases, diminishes with time. There is no great gulf between the social drinker and someone with problems, and some problem drinkers "mature" out of their condition. After age fifty, the percentage of heavy drinkers among women plummets. (Some studies show that men don't have the same huge drop until seventy.)

There is no question, however, that the heavy drinker increases astronomically her chances of becoming alcoholic. In light of this, D. A. Archibald of the Addiction Research Foundation in Canada reports that "as long as we looked upon alcoholics and social drinkers as two entirely separate groups, it was reasonable for us to ignore drinking in general and to concentrate on rehabilitation of alcoholics. But now our studies have shown that these groups are not separate populations. We have been forced to realize that there is no great hope of reducing the numbers of alcoholics or those who drink to levels hazardous to their health without rolling back the overall consumption of alcohol throughout society."

The question of whether only people with peculiar vulnerability to alcohol (either physical or emotional) become alcoholic, no matter what society does, can be debated endlessly. So can the particular sequence of symptoms warning of danger in the future or the presence of the full-blown disease. Nevertheless, what has become clear in the past few years as researchers (many of them women) have looked at the problem is that women are different. They are different both in what leads them to drink too much and in how the disease progresses. Women telescope their drinking history, starting later and progressing faster from heavy drinking into alcoholism. They may even become alcoholic after their mid-forties, a rarity among men.[3] They are more likely to be spree drinkers than steady guzzlers (although there is conflicting evidence), and they drink alone, usually at home (which is where most of them are most of the day). The isolation of women who drink too much is striking—even those on Skid Row don't drink with others. They may, according to Dr. Edith Gomberg "very well be the most isolated and disaffiliated residents." [4] Women's drinking problems seem to be concentrated among those in their thirties and forties; among men, the trouble comes earlier. This may be because men usually start drinking heavily with other men, while women more often get involved later, after marriage, and are more likely to "catch" alcoholism from their drinking husbands than vice versa. For women, it is a contagious disease; teen-age girls, too, are more susceptible than boys to peer pressures to start drinking hard liquor. One bar regular ruefully recalled that she and her husband reflected this pattern: "I started coming here to keep him out of trouble, and now I am as fond of the stuff as he is." Women not only play follow-the-leader in drinking, they are more likely than men to be addicted to other drugs (usually legal ones). The director of an inpatient clinic says, "They come in here with a fistful of pills."

In her article, "Symptoms of Alcoholism in Women," researcher Jane E. James took a first look at women members of AA. She picked up these other differences in the early-warning stage of alcoholism: the women reported personality changes; they (unlike the men) said that heavy drinking was worse for women than for men; forty-three of the eighty-nine women questioned reported they drank more just before or during their menstrual periods; they were supersensitive; and they felt more intelligent and capable when drinking. (One young divorcée revealed her beginning problem at a party when she said, "You wouldn't like me if I hadn't had a few drinks. I'm dull and quiet and uninteresting.") Like the men, women reported increased tolerance ("I'm always the one to drive people home. I can drink anybody under the table.") and an unwillingness to talk about their drinking. The memory blackouts reported by men at this prealcoholic stage didn't turn up for women until the early stages of alcoholism, and downing a drink before a party and guilt about drinking were middle-stage symptoms, not early ones, for the women. The only serious sign that showed up earlier for women than for men was binge drinking. For the most part, the standard early danger signs—gulping drinks, sneaking them—did not appear in women until they hit "bottom." At that point, they started carrying liquor in their purses.

This has some interesting implications for identifying the female problem drinker. If the symptoms are different at different stages for women and for men, diagnoses based on criteria that have been developed for men may be inaccurate or even misleading. The do-it-yourself quizzes—"three yes answers and you are an alcoholic"—may be equally invalid. Even the generalizations about the different course of the disease in men and women have to be accepted with caution. They apply, for the most part, to middle-class women. Psychiatrist Marc Schuckit, who has studied a wide spectrum of female alcoholics, observes, "It appears that lower-status alcoholic women have drinking patterns and drinking problems quite similar to those reported for the average alcoholic male, while higher-status women more closely fit the stereotype in the literature of alcoholism among females." [5]

Since almost everything that is known about women and alcoholism is based on studies of middle-class white women, what follows applies to this group and not necessarily to blue-collar, black, Hispanic, lower-class, or Native American women.

Who are these middle-class women alcoholics? Mercedes McCambridge described her sister sufferers this way: "Three to five percent of us are on skid row. That's all. We are among *you*. . . . We alcoholic women are on the best-dressed lists, the most-admired list year after year. We are social butterflies, the witty darlings of the 'in-group.' We hold office. We sit as judges. We have admirable families. We teach Sunday school. We drive car pools. We offer you coffee, tea, or milk on airplanes and we inject vital serum into your veins. And we are dying by leaps and bounds compared to the rest of you."

In an attempt to separate some of the differences among women themselves, as well as between men and women, Dr. Ruth Fox, a pioneer in the field, has postulated two kinds of alcoholism: primary, which starts early in life, and secondary, which starts late, often after some sort of crisis.

Marge knew that she and alcohol were meant for each other when she was in college. "My mind and drinking got along. I was at my best for a while. For the first time I felt 'finished.' Something had been missing before." Marge is a primary alcoholic.

Helen never drank at all until she was twenty-five. She started drinking heavily in her late thirties after her oldest daughter was killed in an automobile accident "and my life fell apart." She is a secondary alcoholic.

In looking at the life histories of women alcoholics, Dr. Schuckit discovered that this early start/late start distinction was useful in separating women whose drinking coincided with or followed a bout of depression from those who were alcoholic without this complicating psychological factor. Women who become alcoholic later in life are much more likely to suffer from depression along with their abusive drinking than are men, and Dr. Schuckit warns that in women, at least, "Alcoholism may not be a single disease." Sometimes the deep depression preceded the heavy drinking, sometimes it coincided with it. He isn't talking about the "blues" that hit everyone once in a while. He means a deep, pervasive helplessness that can sometimes lead to suicide.

Statistically speaking, Dr. Schuckit writes in *The Archives of Environmental Health* that the typical alcoholic woman is "a forty-five-year-old white woman who began drinking at about age thirty, has about a 50 percent chance of having another psychiatric illness, she is divorced (about 40 percent have been divorced at least once or separated), has attempted suicide (as many as 33 percent have done so in the various studies) and will demonstrate alcoholic withdrawal symptoms with 50 percent probability." Despite Dr. Schuckit's convincing finding, the drug lithium, used to treat depression, has not yet been studied as a treatment possibility for women alcoholics. In men, the results have been equivocal.

Statistics, of course, have very little to do with individuals. They summarize broad patterns and may or may not apply in a particular case. As individuals, instead of as percentages, alcoholic women come from all walks of life and are young, old, successes, and failures.

There is the *successful career woman* who would never make a lunch date. She drank her lunch alone in a dimly lighted bar, then fell asleep with her head on her typewriter in the afternoon. "But I always got my copy in," she says proudly.

One *young divorced mother* tells of waiting until the children got off to school, then going out and buying two six-packs of beer (although beer drinking is not typical of women). "I'd be sure to be mellow when they came home. Instead of screaming I'd be the perfect mother by the time the school bus arrived."

A *suburban housewife* (the category seized on by the popular press as the woman most likely to be alcoholic, although there is no support for this in the studies) says, "I was a bedroom drinker. I'd read, fantasize in bed. My husband lived on TV dinners and Instant Breakfast, but he never complained. He protected me."

The *wealthy woman* often is protected by her money and social position from the recognition that she, too, is abusing alcohol. The daughter of one of them reports, "I'm sure my mother is an alcoholic. She has a drink at the country club at lunch, a few more when she plays bridge, then something when my father comes home. She always has a drink in her hand—vodka, because she thinks it doesn't smell. There are no kids around and a maid to do the work. And my mother is always a lady."

The Gray Panthers organization of *older people* recently became aware of the problem in their age group. One English study by Drs. Arnold J. Rosin and M. M. Glatt estimates that for those over sixty-five, the male/female alcoholism rates are 2:3 in contrast to the general rate of 3:1. It found that more older women than men abused alcohol. They often started drinking heavily in their forties, when they were widowed. What is known about aged Americans and alcohol doesn't fit those statistics—one study doesn't make a trend. But no one doubts that alcoholism can strike older women, too. Among them is the grandmother whose daughter no longer lets her baby-sit. "After she has a few drinks before dinner there may not be any dinner. Once she fell asleep on the couch and the kids were still up when we came home."

Wives of important men may succumb to the disease, too. Marianne Brickley, once the wife of a lieutenant governor of Michigan, said "As my husband climbed the ladder to political success, I stood still. The only thing I changed was my drinking." She felt left out of his busy life and found "the magic potion—alcohol."

There is also an apparent increase in *young people* who become alcoholic, with a growing number of AA groups especially for them. One fourteen-year-old high school girl and AA member recalls, "When I was twelve, everybody was drinking beer. I used to try to drink it too, because I didn't want to spoil the fun. It made me sick. It took a long time before I could drink enough."

Although their lives have been different, all these alcoholic women have three things in common: For a while, alcohol was the magic elixir—it worked; they now abuse the drug; and they have been subjected all their lives to mixed messages about drinking that have made their use of alcohol a greater source of inner conflict than it is for men. Sociologists looking at alcohol use in various cultures have found that the ones with the most problems are the ones with the most conflicting standards for what is acceptable. "Perhaps," psychologist Joan Curlee writes, "there is no group for whom the social signals regarding drinking behavior have been so mixed as for women." One set of signals says drinking is not ladylike. The other set says drinking shows you're mature, sophisticated, and up to date. The relative strength of each message depends, of course, on the woman's religious attachment, education, and socioeconomic group.

Despite all the attention paid to alcoholism in the past decade, no one yet knows what causes it, in either women or men. However, studies on women repeatedly show certain factors in the backgrounds of those who become alcoholic. This repetition doesn't necessarily equal truth; many of the studies were poorly controlled, done on small numbers, and at best are hints of the road future research should take. Any look at a condition as complex as this has to take into account innumerable variables. It is impossible to keep track of them, and this human complexity may lead to well-meaning but false conclusions.

When trying to sort out what is known from what is conjecture, it is a good idea to remember the story of the researchers who found the female hormone estrogen in hops, one of the ingredients of beer. "Beer may be the only drink that can truly enhance a woman's femininity," they reported. It was only later they discovered they hadn't known all the variables. The hops contained estrogen because the women who picked them urinated on them!

With that caveat, some of the evidence about what causes (or is associated with) alcoholism in women can be looked at. The important factors fall roughly into these seven categories.

Alcoholism Runs in Families

Every study that has looked into this question shows that women with a mother, father, sister, or brother who is alcoholic are at much greater risk for developing the disease. One estimate is that the daughter of an alcoholic is three to five times more likely to become alcoholic herself. Young women drug abusers also tend to have alcoholic parents.

Mercedes McCambridge found alcoholics on both sides of her family. Another sober alcoholic, now a counselor, recalls: "My father was an alcoholic although he was never diagnosed as one. I remember seeing him early one morning belting down a drink and holding onto the kitchen table to keep from shaking."

Does the fact that alcoholism runs in families mean the disease is inherited? The evidence is still accumulating. Psychiatrist Donald W. Goodwin did a pioneering study on Danish children born of alcoholics but adopted soon after birth into nonalcoholic families. These were compared with adopted children whose parents had not been hospitalized for alcoholism. The researchers found that the sons of alcoholic men were four times more likely to be alcoholic than the other adopted children, even when they had been brought up in homes where drinking was not a problem. These findings have since been confirmed by others. "The father's sins," Dr. Goodwin concluded, "may be visited upon the sons even in the father's absence." Clearly heredity and not environment was implicated.

The trouble came when the daughters of alcoholics were looked at. To the surprise of the researchers, these young women had no more problems with alcohol than the adoptees from "normal homes," although both had alcoholism rates higher than that of the average Danish woman. Does this mean that the numbers were just too small to draw any conclusions? Could they have missed some alcoholic parents in the control group? Or is alcoholism in some way sex-linked genetically, so that men and not women are more vulnerable? No one knows.

Another hint that there may be a genetic factor comes from Finnish studies. Dr. Juha Partanen and his associates found when comparing identical and fraternal male twins that there was a hereditary component in such traits as amount consumed at any one time, frequency, and abstinence. But they didn't find that identical twins shared an inability to control their drinking, a record of arrests for drunkenness, or social complications due to drinking. Studies on 850 pairs of same-sex twins in this country confirm these findings. Dr. John C. Loehlin mailed detailed questionnaires to twins who participated in the National Merit Scholarship exams and found identical twins were much more alike than fraternal twins in their drinking patterns. There was, he concluded, "an appreciable genetic involvement in heavy drinking, but little involvement in other aspects of alcohol use."

This, of course, brings us back to what alcoholism is. Certainly no one is suggesting that the social symptoms of the condition—including automobile accidents, difficulties on the job—are passed on from one generation to another, but in men, at least, the propensity for heavy drinking seems to be. This is a clue that there may be a predisposing physical factor involved. There are also the people who feel sick or headachey after drinking only small amounts or who, like many Orientals, flush uncomfortably. These people, through no virtue of their own, may be genetically protected from alcoholism, just as those who can tolerate large amounts may be genetically more vulnerable. There is also evidence from studies of identical twins in this country that the rate at which alcohol is metabolized may be inherited; some people may get drunk faster and stay drunk longer than others.[6]

A general caution about genetic studies in this complex area was sounded by Dr. Morris Chafetz when he wrote: "There are two dangers in the heredity theory. First, it reinforces the widespread and unjustified sense of futility about trying to treat alcoholic people. Second, by insisting on a hereditary factor, we introduce that strong barrier of hope and change, the self-fulfilling prophecy." If you expect something to happen, you will act consciously or unconsciously, to make it happen.

There is some evidence that the family atmosphere, rather than genes, may play a more significant part for women alcoholics. They report more early parental deaths than men do and more family problems. Dr. Edith Gomberg sums it up with, "We believe that there are kinds of disruptive early experiences—families in which divorce, death, desertion, alcoholism, psychiatric illness occur—and that these produce a vulnerable person, a woman who has great difficulty in trusting others." This woman finds, however, that she can trust the bottle—always available, quick to act, never rejecting. She may also have learned from an alcoholic parent that drinking is the way to cope with stress. A teen-aged alcoholic remembered that her hard-drinking mother offered her some sherry when she came home from junior high school complaining that her teachers were awful, the work was too hard, her friends unbearable. She soon found herself drinking whenever things got rough.

A woman who comes from a large family also runs a greater risk of alcoholism, although it isn't as great as it is for men. And, if she is the youngest of the brood, her chances of trouble increase. The guess is that large families may mean "diluted parenting" or may reflect ethnic differences that also seem to predispose to alcoholism. As for the baby in the family, she may get used to being pampered, increasing her expectation of instant gratification, first by a bottle with milk, later by one with alcohol.[7]

Women Alcoholics Are Particularly Vulnerable to Life Crises

In 1969, psychologist Joan Curlee, who had worked with alcoholics at the Hazelden Foundation in Minneapolis, published an article about women there. She called it "Alcoholism and the 'Empty Nest.'" Since that time, other researchers have found that women alcoholics often say they began drinking heavily after a divorce, widowhood, menopause, or the time the last child left home. It is not clear whether some hormonal changes in midlife make a woman who has not been previously addicted especially vulnerable to alcohol; what is clear is that thirty out of the hundred responsible, well-put-together, middle-class women Dr. Curlee studied "blamed" their excessive drinking on a painful personal event. Only eight of the hundred men did. Often, the drinking that started fairly late in life quickly escalated into alcoholism.

Dr. Curlee told the story of a middle-aged woman whose husband had been a topflight city official for more than a quarter of a century. She prided herself on being "Mr. X's wife." When he lost his job, she began drinking heavily. Although he soon started his own successful business, she could never recapture her old social position and felt shut out of his new, busy life.

Three other women whose problems escalated within a nine-month period were single parents with only children. When the nest emptied, they were left without a reason for living.

For all these women, the trauma had something to do with a change in their roles as wives and mothers, a change that shook

their already fragile sense of womanliness. As Dr. Curlee poignantly writes, "The question 'Who am I?' is difficult at age fifteen;
it is excruciating at age fifty."

Even at other times, women who are not necessarily alcoholic
are likely to blame their excessive drinking on something that has
upset them. When police in a northern California county arrested
ninety people for drunken driving in a three-month period, they
asked them what had happened just before they were picked up.
Of the thirty women, twenty-nine could point to something specific. Only half the men could. This may reflect society's standards,
since women are supposed to be less able to withstand stress. Men
are supposed to be stoical. In her usual sensible way, Dr. Gomberg
questions the findings of a series of studies which include as wide-
ranging a list of crises as can be found in a year of soap operas.
"Women give a stressful incident more often than men," she says,
"but is it that women are more defensive? You can always find a
trauma—the coffee pot boiled over so I drank—but are women
really more vulnerable to stress or more defensive?"

Elizabeth Morrissey and Marc Schuckit, while at the University
of Washington, suggested that the women who give a precipitating incident may be reacting to the way the question is asked,
rather than to the way things really happened. Carefully structured interviews of almost 200 lower-class women admitted to a
Seattle detoxification center showed that most of them had had
their first symptoms of problem drinking a year before a classic
stressful event (menopause, divorce) or three years afterwards—
not in a "my divorce drove me to drink" pattern. The interviewers
were careful to separate questions about the onset of heavy drinking from questions about miscarriages or divorce, "thus discouraging the subjects from using one life problem as an explanation for
the occurrence of another."

Sex-Role Conflicts

Some alcoholic women feel insecure as women. This uneasiness
about their feminine identity may play a part in the gynecological
difficulties they report and in their heavier use of alcohol just before or during a menstrual period.

When she studied the medical histories of alcoholic and nonalcoholic women, psychologist Sharon Wilsnack found a striking dif-

ference in the incidence of obstetrical disorders. Seventy-eight percent of the alcoholic women, but only 8 percent of the nonalcoholics, had had obstetrical or gynecological problems, and these had occurred before drinking became a problem. Did a conflict about their abilities as women play a part in precipitating the troubles? Did this "malfunctioning" in a woman's role lead to excessive drinking? The questions are provocative, the answers still obscure. But when menopause or other assaults on her feminine identity hit her, this confused woman may "begin a vicious circle, with the typical consequences of heavy drinking—e.g., neglect of appearance, disapproval of family and friends—posing new threats to her sense of feminine adequacy. The new threats can cause her to drink even more heavily, until her nondrinking alternatives for feeling womanly are severely restricted and she becomes completely dependent on alcohol."

Dr. Wilsnack also points out that this sex-role conflict may show itself clearly only after marriage; women who become alcoholic tend to marry at the same rates as others, but have higher rates of divorce, separation, and desertion. Given her uncertainty about her femininity, "Marriage, children, and the inevitable frustrations and stresses lead this vulnerable woman toward problem drinking." [8]

Although members of this group see themselves as womanly, they have conflicts and anxieties about how well they can do the jobs traditionally assigned to their sex—being a good wife and mother. They are the women who outwardly value femininity but inwardly have strong masculine attitudes. When Dr. Wilsnack tested alcoholic women she found they answered questions about whether they like to cook and whether men have more opportunities than women just as nonalcoholic women did. On the question of importance of motherhood, they were even more "feminine" than the control group. Yet unconsciously they had hidden "masculine" traits; they scored a lot more like men on a true-false test that measured their assertiveness. Dr. Wilsnack conjectures that these women may have had aggressive or assertive personal styles that didn't fit their own conception of what a woman should be. They accepted the stereotype but couldn't live up to it. Drinking, she says, may have made them feel more feminine and closer to their own ideal self-images. When they were young they may have managed without alcohol, but as life went on and they were faced with gynecological difficulties, divorce, or widowhood, their sense of themselves as less than adequate intensified; the "empty nest" syndrome of problem drinking in midlife may be one attempt to deal with this inner sex-role conflict.[9]

Another study of one hundred alcoholic women described them as "hyperfeminine," but with "competitive emasculating" lifestyles. Again, these are women who are somewhat masculine in the aggressive way they deal with life, but play the part of the eyelash-batting, helpless female on the surface. And in one of the few looks at alcoholic wives (there have been many looks at wives of alcoholic husbands), their husbands, who saw beyond the façade, described them as dominating and competitive—the masculine style again.[10]

This kind of woman's adolescence is summed up by Dr. Edith Gomberg this way: "As the mating season begins, she joins the game with intensity and she is OVERTLY, on the surface, a very feminine young lady. Under the hyperfemininity is a resentful young woman. This *conflict about sexual role* is so striking it has been observed in four different, independent observations."

These are the women who psychiatrist Howard P. Wood of Philadelphia said had the "Magnolia Blossom syndrome." Most of the subjects he studied had been brought up in the South and were attractive, stylish, and womanly, yet they felt miserably inadequate—decorative but useless. They had never been able to satisfy the dominant figure in their lives—their mother.

One therapist who has worked with alcoholics says life for some of his comparable women patients was a Shirley Temple act. "Their mothers dressed them in curls and ruffles and they were put on display. But although they never got angry or dirty, they were never doll-like enough. They felt they weren't seen as real people; that a part of themselves had to be kept hidden."

Another kind of sex-role conflict that may operate in some alcoholic women is illustrated by Bobbie, in her third month at a halfway house. She consciously rejects the feminine stereotypes (like Annie Oakley, "anything you can do I can do better"), yet she feels herself trapped by society's requirements that she be a wife, mother, and dutiful daughter. Since 1970, researchers have been finding this pattern more and more often. Perhaps, some speculate, it is a reflection of the women's movement, which has called on women to be more competitive and assertive, less bound by traditional, nurturing rules. Outwardly, Bobbie thinks this is the way things should be; inwardly, she is as much a product of the "sugar and spice and everything nice" picture of little girls as her hyperfeminine counterpart.

The trouble with both groups is that they are bound by society's expectations and have had to deny or squelch a side of themselves—the "expressive" side if they consciously value "masculinity," the "assertive" side if they consciously value "femininity." Drinking may offer them a way of getting the two opposing sides to blend into harmony. Or, using Dr. Wilsnack's formulation, the alcohol may flood them with feminine feelings, allowing them time out from the painful conflict.

Just how much this conflict contributes to alcoholism is not clear. There are those who argue that in our society the day of androgyny has not yet come, and that most women (and men, too) feel themselves forced to deny one side or another of their personalities. Yet only a small percentage resort to alcohol to cope with the stress. Who they are may depend on the strength of this conflict and its interaction with other predisposing factors. The hope is that as assertive women and supportive men become more acceptable, sex-role conflicts will diminish and so, perhaps, will alcohol abuse.

The classic Freudian-based view is that alcoholism is a defense against homosexual feelings. One would expect, then, that the active homosexual might have less need for it, but tentative, small-scale research on lesbians indicates that they have higher rates of alcoholism than heterosexual women. They also have consequences of heavy drinking, such as car accidents and arrests, that strongly resemble the trouble patterns of men. In Los Angeles, a survey of the gay community by Lillene Fifield came up with an estimate that 25-35 percent of all gays were alcoholic.[11] Dr. Wilsnack found that all ten lesbians she studied became more aggressive and assertive, physically as well as verbally, when they drank—another pattern of behavior that fits the male stereotype.

A Possible Physical Basis for Alcoholism

The first solid experimental evidence that some chemical quirk in the alcoholic's brain may make him or her drink came in 1977 with a report on rats who normally reject alcohol. When neurobiologists Robert Myers and Christine Melchoir of Purdue University injected a substance into the rats' brains, animals who had previously scorned ethyl alcohol and preferred water began lapping up the alcohol. After a while, the rats even began showing symptoms of alcoholism, including a rodent version of delirium tremens (the D.T.'s) involving whisker twitching and "wet-dog shakes."

The substance the researchers injected—tetrahydropapaveroline (THP)—is part of the metabolic process that breaks down alcohol in the body. What this suggests, according to Dr. Myers, is that alcoholics may differ from other people in that their brains store THP after they drink, and this then propels them into more drinking. The report states: "We now present evidence that if THP is present in the brain of a rat for a protracted period of time, the animal will drink excessive amounts of alcohol in a free-choice situation where water is also available. If that is the case, the analogy would hold for the human."

Even after nine months without alcohol, the rats preferred alcohol to water—an indication that abstention does not alter the mechanism once it has been established, and a warning that alcohol may continue to be dangerous for anyone who has had a drinking problem. There is a possibility that some way may be found to alter brain chemistry, eliminate the excess THP, and help the alcoholic stop drinking.

Another useful finding has come as the side result of a study of cirrhosis of the liver and may result in a precise way to identify alcoholics without depending on fuzzy definitions or inaccurate drinking histories. Certain substances in the blood of baboons given heavy alcohol doses were found to persist even after the alcohol had disappeared from their bloodstreams. When the test was tried on alcoholics, the two telltale amino acids (protein building blocks) could be recovered, even a week after drinking had stopped, in double the quantity found in control subjects who didn't drink. The researchers—Drs. Spencer Shaw, Barry Stimmel, and Charles Lieber of New York—don't know why this is so. But they hope their test and an understanding of the process by which it works will be useful in identifying heavy drinkers, predicting who might become alcoholic, and helping to identify those who have an especially high risk of developing cirrhosis of the liver. "At the moment," Dr. Lieber cautions, "the test is not a predictor of who will become a heavy drinker but a determinant of who is a heavy drinker."

Dr. Henry Rosett of Boston City Hospital has experimented with it for this purpose, trying to identify women coming to a prenatal clinic as heavy drinkers and help them stop drinking, using the threat of damage to the fetus as a powerful motivation. Reports by the women themselves of how much they drink are notoriously inaccurate; this simple blood test could turn up hidden heavy drinkers before it is too late for their unborn children. (See chapter 9, "Alcohol and Pregnancy.")

These studies are, of course, just the beginning of an understanding of what may be a physical component in alcoholism. There is still the question of whether some kind of hormonal imbalance in women might be associated with both gynecological problems (which many alcoholic women report) and a particular sensitivity to alcohol. (See chapter 6, "For Women Only.")

For years, some alcoholics have been echoing Mercedes McCambridge: "Biochemically, I am convinced I was born an alcoholic." Social scientists and some physicians have been equally convinced that what is known up to now does not support this view. Dr. Morris Chafetz writes: "People always ask, 'What about the person who takes one drink and is a confirmed alcoholic?' I have heard these stories, too, and a few patients have reported that this was their history. But I also know that if an Orthodox Jewish rabbi were eating some meat and you informed him it was meat from a pig, he would have a physiological response . . . yet I can't conceive that there is a metabolic defect in Orthodox Jews that causes a reaction to pork products. So, yes, I can imagine certain combinations of physical, psychological, and cultural experiences that would produce an unusual response to the first drink—a response that could label someone as an alcoholic from the first drink. But it wouldn't be the alcohol that did it, and such a response would be very rare indeed."

Dr. Chafetz may be right. But a new study indicates that there *is* something different about the way an alcoholic's body reacts to alcohol, and this may be connected with addiction and the physical damage that often results. In their continuing studies, Dr. Charles Lieber and his associates in the Bronx found that acetaldehyde (a powerful metabolic product of alcohol) reaches a higher level in alcoholics, and stays there longer, than it does in social drinkers, even when the two groups have the same blood-alcohol levels. It isn't clear yet whether the difference precedes or follows the alcoholism. But the buildup of acetaldehyde may account for some of alcohol's damage to vital organs and suggests that some basic physical difference may be part of the explanation of why some drinkers become alcoholic and others do not.

More information may come from brain-wave studies that show young sons of alcoholics—even before they have begun to drink— with certain patterns that mimic those of heavy drinkers. These studies have led some researchers to divide alcoholics into two basic groups—familial (those with a genetic tendency) and nonfamilial.

There Is No Alcoholic Personality

All sorts of women become addicted to this drug. But there are certain psychological patterns that show up again and again in the personalities of women alcoholics; they also show up in the life histories of women who have other emotional disorders. Psychologist Linda Beckmann thinks it possible that "the few traits such as depression, neuroticism, and poor self-esteem that often appear in alcoholic women are characteristic of most women with emotional problems and that the only special characteristic of alcoholic women is that they misuse alcohol."

Nevertheless, alcoholic women are often described as needing immediate gratification, overly dependent ("they believe, and parrot back, whatever anyone tells them," one counselor complained), orally fixated (so that heavy drinkers tend to be heavy smokers, too), and immature. Since most of the studies were done on women who were already alcoholic, carrying the crushing burden of guilt that society (and the woman herself) heaps on the woman who drinks too much, it is impossible to tell which of these characteristics led to drinking, and which followed it.

A clue may come from a long-term study that makes it possible to look back at the adolescent personalities of women now in their forties and fifties. Middle-class, white, Oakland, California, girls who later turned out to be problem drinkers were seen in their junior and senior high school days as self-defeating, lacking in charm, vulnerable, withdrawn, and sensitive to criticism—in other words, girls who didn't think very highly of themselves. The startling thing is that these same characteristics were shared with women who, in middle age, were abstainers. But the adult abstainers were more responsible, ethical, and emotionally controlled. Dr. Mary C. Jones found that the problem drinkers, in contrast, were submissive as youngsters, but rebellious as adults. Those who became moderate drinkers were the girls who were likable and who liked themselves. Although the numbers were small, the study suggests that character traits evident as early as the eighth grade may play a part in later drinking patterns, and that difficulties in coping and low self-esteem may be associated with problem drinking or staying away from alcohol completely in later life.

As for the depression that often rides in tandem with heavy drinking, some of it is a result of alcohol which has, for centuries, been noted for its ability to unstopper the flow of tears. But Dr. Marc Schuckit has found that a deeper kind of depression, which psychiatrists call "affective disorder," is part of the prealcoholic history of 25–30 percent of the women he studied. These women had been almost totally incapacitated by their severe depression—an "affective disorder"—and usually started drinking heavily after a psychiatric hospitalization (other alcoholic women, he found, drink at the same time as the episode of severe depression). Twenty-five percent of the mothers and sisters of these women had this kind of psychiatric illness, too. The drinking, then, was probably a symptom of an underlying disease and different from the kind of drinking that starts earlier and is a disease in itself. The mothers and sisters of these early-onset women were more likely to be alcoholic without severe depression.

Suicide is a risk for both alcoholics and those suffering from affective disorders, but it is most likely to occur in women who show both severe problems. Paradoxically, hospitalization for a suicide attempt seems to make a woman more open to treatment than hospitalization for other complications of alcoholism.

One mother and career woman drank only socially for twenty years even though she had suffered from depressions since adolescence. After her first child was born, she sank into a severe postpartum depression, but didn't increase her alcohol consumption. Her compulsive drinking started only after another emotional low point—a bout with the mumps. Eventually addicted to both barbiturates and alcohol (double addiction is more typical of women than of men), she tried suicide—and, true to the pattern uncovered in Dr. Schuckit's studies, was then finally open to successful treatment.

The low self-esteem that haunts alcoholic women of both types has been examined by Harvard psychologist Howard T. Blane. He found that "the central, perhaps inevitable feature ... is a concern, even a preoccupation, about being inadequate and inept. . . . Obviously, depression is often the dominant and complicating emotional accompaniment." These feelings sometimes become unbearable, he noticed, when women face marriage or the necessity of moving from college to the world of work. "The idea of the unfulfilled promise and the despairing sense of ineptness go hand in hand." The world has seemed a wonderful place with happiness there for the taking, but real life doesn't quite live up to these dreams.

Dr. Gomberg followed these feelings into marriage, noting "No marriage can possibly live up to the fantasies of our vulnerable, hyperfeminine young lady. Sometimes, when the marriage fails, she goes out and finds a job—and starts drinking there. Sometimes she stays home and drinks. . . . She finds in alcohol a friend who is a) always there, always dependable; b) available when she wants it without delay; c) a source of disturbance to people around her—it gets everyone annoyed and upset and worried and angry. With that potent weapon to fight back at a frustrating world, it is a wonder we don't have more women alcoholics than we do." Women who abuse alcohol have found that it works—it does what they want it to do.

Alcoholic men have been seen as overly dependent, but having to disguise it; since women in our society can be dependent more openly, they may be protected from the need to use alcohol quite as much. Black women, however, who have to assume the role of family provider more often, cannot afford dependency and are reported to have a rate of alcoholism that closely approaches that of black men.

No One Can Predict Who Will Become Alcoholic

It would be nice if the experts could say, "You ninety women can go home and drink whatever you like, when you like, and nothing will happen to you. You ten had better watch out for problems." (An estimated 10 percent of all drinkers become alcoholic.) But it isn't that clearcut. Alcoholism is obviously a complex disorder with physical, social, and cultural components.

Nevertheless, long-term studies indicate that personal characteristics in adolescence, before drinking began, and drinking patterns in college may signal later problems. The Oakland Growth Study, as we have seen, suggests that adolescent girls who lack some of the social graces and think very little of themselves may run a higher risk of becoming problem drinkers later in life.

And in a second look at a study that was done in 1949 on thousands of college students, sociologist Kaye Fillmore, then of the Rutgers Center for Alcohol Studies, found that drinking habits in college could predict trouble twenty years later. The warning signs, though, were different for men and for women, and it was easier to predict for men. "Symptomatic drinking"—drinking before a party, suffering memory blackouts, taking one or more drinks before or instead of breakfast, getting one or two drinks ahead of everyone else without noticing it—was the best predictor of problems in later life for women. Binge drinking in college didn't turn up in the histories of those women who later had trouble, but it was very important as a predictor for men.

Women who drank for the age-old reasons of relieving fatigue or tension, forgetting a disappointment, or coping with a crisis also were more likely to abuse alcohol later on. "In fact," Dr. Fillmore says, "one might suggest that early alcohol problems are more 'serious' in terms of the future among women than among men." This may be due to cultural attitudes which add extra weight to a woman's guilt and self-loathing.

There were other categories of women who ran into trouble with alcohol in their forties and fifties: those who dropped out of college and also showed symptomatic drinking; those who married below the educational and social status of their own families; and women whose early lives had a lot of change and inconsistency. For both men and women, moving up the social and economic ladder was the best single protection against problem drinking.

Dr. Fillmore also prefers "problem drinking" to "alcoholism," and says the two are not synonymous. Using Dr. Cahalan's criteria of seven problem areas, she says, "We're having a lot of trouble with the women. We can't find many of them. We've found just 8 percent of our women are problem drinkers, as against 16 percent of the men. I can't explain it. Women are certainly drinking, but they seem to be drinking socially. This study hasn't turned up figures to match the concern about women approaching men in problem drinking. From what we've seen, alcoholism is not on the upswing among middle- and upper-class women in their forties and fifties."

What the outlook for the future will be, no one can predict. Figures on teen-agers (Dr. Fillmore says she can't speak for younger women) with drinking patterns approaching that of boys may indicate that a follow-up study done twenty years from now will show different predictors and different problem rates.

Social Forces Contribute to Alcoholism

It's clear that genetic and psychological factors play a part in who becomes alcoholic. So do what sociologists call "orienting factors"—attitudes that make drinking acceptable and situations that make alcohol readily available to the woman who tends to use it to satisfy her emotional needs.

Urban women and those who have at least some college are exposed to an atmosphere that makes drinking socially acceptable. Often, too, the college woman learns her drinking patterns early from men friends.

Working women are slightly more likely than the stay-at-home to become alcoholic; one industry treatment program turned up a 13 percent incidence in contrast to the 8 percent estimate of alcoholic women in the general population. This may, of course, be a reflection of the fact that women at work are less able to hide their problem. It may also be a warning that women in management positions, at least, run a higher risk. Karen Zuckerman, formerly in charge of New York State's programs for women alcoholics in industry, says the executive woman is exposed to the rituals of power—business lunches, cocktails—and "unless she's careful she learns to equate alcohol prowess with success."

"Careless drinking" is another danger in social groups which accept alcohol as one of the good things in life. Dr. Vernon Johnson, author of *I'll Quit Tomorrow*, tells of the "sip, sip, sip" of weekend homeowners who start to unwind as soon as they get to their vacation home Friday evening and keep it up at a party or barbecue until late Sunday night. "Then," he says, "they sleep it off because they know they shouldn't drive and they go back to the city on Monday morning."

In a broader look at what is behind the social drinking that slips into problem drinking, sociologist Don Cahalan found in his national study that the person who has good things to say about drinking and enjoys getting drunk once in a while is most likely to be a problem drinker.

Ethnic differences, of course, play a part in developing and perpetuating these attitudes. So do social and economic position. And sociologists have noticed that as women approach men in the roles they play in society, they approach men in drinking practices—and problems—too. The same was true in ancient times. One of the archaeological finds of Egypt's seventeenth dynasty is this exultant command by an upper-class woman: "Give me eighteen cups of wine, behold I should love drunkenness." A few hundred years later, at about the time of Tutankhamen, an artist immortalized another woman's drunkenness in a tomb painting showing a banquet guest leaning forward in misery and a servant running with a vase to catch her vomit. She missed. But the fact that the scene was worth preserving for the afterlife attests to the popularity of overindulgence, particularly for women. They were the equals of men in other, more enviable, things, too. The German scholar F. Max Müller wrote, "No people, ancient or modern, has given women so high a legal status as did the inhabitants of the Nile Valley."

In addition to equal legal rights and equal rights to get drunk, the ancient Greek historian Herodotus credited Egyptian women with following "exactly the reverse of the common practice of mankind. . . . The women attend the market and trade while the men sit at home at the loom. . . . Women stand up to urinate, men sit down . . . sons need not support their parents unless they choose, but daughters must, whether they choose or no." The Greek historian's modern editor couldn't resist this skeptical note: "he [Herodotus] has indulged in the marvelous at the sacrifice of truth." But the truth is, as sociologist Viola Mannheim puts it, "The more of the formerly masculine functions women fulfill, the more of those traits previously thought 'masculine' they generally develop."

Brenda McLeod, a twenty-two-year-old native of New York City, found herself in a classic situation illustrating how masculine

roles and drinking go together. Unhappy in her deck job on a tug-
boat pushing Navy vessels around, she was asked how she happened to be in such a fix. In the time-honored response of sailors
all over the world, she answered: "I was drunk. I got out of the
army and was partying with some friends. We all got drunk, and
they talked me into enlisting in the Navy."

Have our own changing social roles propelled more women into
alcoholism as well as into social drinking? The women's movement
is often singled out as the villain but, as Dr. Gomberg sensibly
points out, "There is, in fact, a lot of disagreement as to whether
the emancipation of women LESSENS or MAGNIFIES the extent
of alcoholism among them. I don't see how such a question can be
really resolved—it is an emotional issue, complexly tying together
women's rights, changes in patterns of acceptable social behavior,
the dissatisfactions and frustrations of contemporary existence—
and alcohol. But we would be foolish to accept a simple formula.
To say FREE WOMEN FROM KUCHE, KIRCH, KINDER AND
END ALCOHOLISM is as silly as saying that THE EMANCIPA-
TION OF WOMEN LEADS TO ALCOHOLISM AND MORAL
DECAY."

A willowy, red-haired AA member recognized the absurdity of
blaming her drinking on the movement for equality when she told
a meeting in midtown Manhattan: "I kidded myself that I was
striking a blow for women's liberation by going into a bar alone
and sitting on a stool and paying for my own drinks."

The French, too, are caught in conflicting attitudes. One study
concludes that "alcohol represents the ransom woman pays for her
emancipation." Yet statistician Marguerite Bontemps reports that
alcoholism is decreasing among Frenchwomen as they move into
higher status jobs. It is the men who are drinking more under stress
as they lose jobs to the ladies.

Margaret Mead pointed out that getting a job and emancipating
herself from the home may not be the answer for a woman who
runs the risk of increasing her stresses and drinking at work as well
as at home. Yet the woman who stays home may be locked into the
"unfulfilled promise" situation so eloquently described by Dr.
Blane. Jan DuPlain, former director of the National Council on Alcoholism's office on women, affirms what is clear to anyone who
has looked at today's situation of shifting roles: "The answer to

female alcoholism is not going to come by returning women to their former roles."

Ms. DuPlain credits the women's movement with the establishment in 1976 of the office she headed and has dedicated herself to gaining recognition of alcoholism as also a woman's disease. She firmly feels that an alliance between the women's movement and the movement to deal with alcoholism in women is the surest way to a solution to the problem.

Susan B. Anthony, grandniece and namesake of the pioneering suffragette, agrees. She chose the fiftieth anniversary of the date of women's suffrage to announce at a press conference on Capitol Hill that she was a recovered alcoholic. Commandingly tall and as intense as her namesake, she said, "I'm part of two movements— the one in which women were the leading agents for social change, the other in which alcoholics are the primary agents for personal change in our century." She sees AA's self-help method as the precursor of group therapy in the treatment of psychological disorders and the model for women's consciousness raising. She also concedes that as women move into the marketplace, "naturally they will take on the diseases of the working male—hypertension, alcoholism. Naturally the woman under pressure will be tense. But frustration is more likely to lead to alcoholism. Self-expression is not achieved in the house. The hidden housewife's only high comes out of a bottle."

Obviously the question of how much the women's movement has either prevented or increased the misuse of alcohol can never be answered. Certainly the movement has accomplished three things: it has brought women alcoholics more out into the open to seek treatment earlier, recognizing that alcoholism is a woman's disease, too; it has prodded treatment facilities to recognize the special needs of women; and it has put the spotlight on low self-esteem in women—alcoholic as well as the general population— with the conviction that a strong sense of self will help prevent alcohol abuse.

What should a woman do if she is concerned about her own drinking? Problem drinking is as much a matter of attitude as of intake. Even one drink, if it's an absolute must, may signal trouble. Creeping acceleration, too, is something to watch out for. The NIAAA said bluntly in an advertising campaign, "If you have to

have a drink to feel social, that's not social drinking." Dr. Sheila
Blume, who has worked with alcoholics in her private practice as
well as in a state hospital, says: "What you have to do is look at
yourself and your drinking and decide how important it is. Do you
ever feel you just have to go out—even in a storm—to get a bottle
of sherry or vodka because you're used to that one drink to unwind? Why do you need it? Try to reschedule yourself if it's so indispensable. Why do you have so much trouble unwinding? If
you're working try to remove some of the tensions. At home, get a
baby-sitter in the late afternoon so you won't be sitting around
when you usually reach for a drink. Some people use alcohol to
bolster a lifestyle—as a means of adjustment. It helps them handle
things they can't handle. Maybe they're trying to be too perfect.
Maybe they shouldn't try to do too much."

In a similar vein, Dr. Thomas Harford, the social psychologist
whose Boston study turned up definite situational patterns for
drinking, suggests that the woman who is wondering about her intake should keep a diary of her drinking for one week. When?
Where? With whom? How much? Then she may find that lunch
on Friday with Jane is the time she has more than she thinks is
good for her. Maybe she shouldn't make that a regular thing. Or
maybe she should spend more Saturday nights with friends who
drink less than she does. Changing the situation may change the
drinking.

Anyone who has doubts about her own drinking might want to
try Marty Mann's no-nonsense test that has made the situation
clear to many people who were able to dodge reality. Mrs. Mann,
who founded the National Council on Alcoholism, suggested "for
six months at least decide you will stick to a certain number of
drinks a day (not less than one or more than three)—if not daily,
then set the limit for days when you do drink—weekends, for instance. There's no deviance allowed for celebration or consolation,
and absolutely no exceptions or the test has been failed." A shorter
trial time won't work, she said, because many people with problems can control their drinking for a while.

The woman who can't stick to the plan has a clear signal that
she needs help. The earlier in the process treatment starts, the
more successful it is likely to be.

6

For Women Only

Women have been drinking alcohol since the first grapes fermented into wine and the first grain soured and bubbled into beer. But the possibility that we might react differently to this drug because of our unique physiology seems never to have occurred to the scientists who investigated alcohol's effects. Most of the research has been done by men on men—the latter usually alcoholic, usually undernourished. Only in the last decade has science acknowledged that even nice women drink and that we are not just smaller versions of men. It now seems possible that hormonal changes may play a key role in the way alcohol affects women. The evidence is preliminary and sketchy but, as Dr. Edith Gomberg sees it, "We are at the beginning of an understanding that there is a relationship between alcohol, hormonal states, and metabolic functioning."

The unlikely leader in providing this understanding has been a young, black-bearded Oklahoma psychologist. Dr. Ben Morgan Jones did most of his work in the second-floor laboratory of a converted mansion smack in the middle of Oklahoma City, with an oil well pumping a few feet from the door. His work has pinpointed these special effects of alcohol on women:

1. The menstrual cycle affects the way a woman reacts to drinking.[1]
2. Thinking, as measured by reaction time, slows down during key points in the menstrual cycle when a woman drinks.[2]
3. Women get drunk faster than men on equivalent amounts of alcohol.
4. Women on birth-control pills have reactions that resemble men's.
5. "Pudgies"—women with a generous amount of body fat—metabolize alcohol more slowly than "skinnies"—women with a lean body build.[3]

Although many of these effects seem to be related to hormonal levels, the findings are inconclusive because Dr. Jones and his colleagues (one of whom is his wife, Marilyn) have tied their research to their subjects' own reports of menstrual cycles. Having a woman do the interviewing and testing made their subjects feel at ease and increased the likelihood of accurate information, but they did not actually take blood samples to assess what the hormonal level was on any given day.

In his first experiment Dr. Morgan tested twenty women on the first day of menstrual flow, on the intermenstrual day (about the fourteenth, when ovulation presumably occurs), and about the twenty-eighth day—the premenstrual time. The young women were told to fast for four hours before the test, and then were given 1.5 ounces of 198-proof alcohol mixed with orange drink—the equivalent of two stiff drinks, adjusted according to weight. Every five or ten minutes they took a sophisticated "drunk driving" test, blowing into a machine that records approximate blood-alcohol levels from the alcohol that is exhaled. One of them said, "It was like blowing up a whole package of balloons for a kid's party, one after another. It's hard work."

The women became most intoxicated on the premenstrual day, just before their period was to begin; they had their lowest blood-alcohol levels during the flow, and at the midpoint the blood-alcohol levels were at the middle level, too. Dr. Jones uses "intoxicated" instead of "drunk" to avoid confusing social behavior with a scientific measurement. What counts is not how tipsy a person acts, but how much alcohol is in the bloodstream. These results were so startling that he repeated the experiment with another group. He got the same results. Finally he laboriously tested three women every day for a month, having them check basal temperatures each morning to determine the time of ovulation. Here too, it was evident that the biggest jolt from alcohol usually came just before menstruation, the least effect was during the flow, and a middle effect occurred at about the time of ovulation. Dr. Jones readily admits that he hasn't proven that hormonal levels have a direct effect on blood-alcohol levels. He has only been able to approximate what's happening, because in these tests he hadn't done blood tests for hormones, and the menstrual cycle hardly behaves with machinelike regularity. "Like any group data," he cautions, "what we have found may not apply to a particular woman. Our individual studies showed that not every woman necessarily shows her highest peak premenstrually." As a matter of fact, a study in England found that, contrary to Dr. Morgan's early results, there was no variation in peak blood-alcohol levels at different times in the menstrual cycle. These researchers used blood tests to check hormonal levels, but unfortunately they worked with a small sample. The question is still being investigated.[4]

Curious about whether men, too, showed fluctuations in their response to alcohol, Dr. Jones tested three men three times during a span of thirty days—about the way he had tested the women. In sharp contrast to his earlier findings, the men showed remarkable consistency in their blood-alcohol levels. One man tested every week for three months was monotonously predictable in his reactions. As Dr. Jones suggests, "The great variability in response to alcohol in women may make them more cautious when drinking. A woman may obtain a blood alcohol level and feel minimal effects from alcohol on one occasion and then may become very intoxicated and act drunk on another occasion after consuming the same amount of alcohol." Men, on the other hand, can be pretty sure of their limits.

In a look at the effects of alcohol on reaction time during the menstrual cycle, Dr. Jones was surprised to find that, after a drink, women's reactions are slower at all three key points—just before the flow begins, at the midpoint, and during the flow—than they are during the rest of the month. As an indication that hormone levels may have something to do with this too, women on the pill showed this effect only at the point they stop taking the contraceptive—the premenstrual time, when their hormone levels plummet.

But Dr. Alfonso Paredes, who headed the Oklahoma Alcohol Center when the research was done there, has some doubts. "I don't quite believe the effect of alcohol and the menstrual cycle on reaction time," he says. "My guess is that findings of future research are not going to be very striking. Culturally we've attributed more bad things to this biological event than it deserves, and its impact on thinking may have more to do with emotional meaning than with the event itself."

Whatever future research may turn up, Dr. Jones has already confirmed another hallowed canard: As barroom observers have been saying for years, women do get drunk faster than men on equivalent doses of alcohol. Even when he carefully adjusted the alcohol dosage for weight, he found that women reached peak blood-alcohol levels faster. Obviously, it isn't just a matter of size. Probably it has something to do with the fact that men have more water in their tissues than women; the alcohol, then, is more diluted.

Women also get rid of the alcohol faster than men. In practical terms, this means that a woman may be "coming down" when the man she is with is still "getting high." Put her slump and his exhilaration together and the discrepancy may wreck what might have been a lovely evening.

Millions of women on birth-control pills don't have naturally occurring menstrual cycles. Are their reactions different? The answer is both yes and no. Like other women, they reach peak blood-alcohol levels faster than men. But there the sisterly similarity ends. Women on the pill take longer to get rid of the alcohol than other women and thus resemble men in their pattern. This means that the effects of a drink last longer, and one may do the work of two. They will also match their male friends as the evening wears on, reaching the down-curve slump at about the same time.

Women with the slowest rates of alcohol metabolism were what Marilyn Jones called the "pudgies"—those with considerable body fat for their height. Pudgies on the pill took longest to get the alcohol out of their systems. The "skinnies" off the pill had the fastest rate, perhaps indicating that lean women not taking birth-control pills can drink more with less effect.

The differences between women menstruating normally and those whose cycle has been interfered with by artificial hormones lead to some interesting questions. Researchers have noticed that rats given estrogens or oral contraceptives cut down on their intake of alcohol voluntarily. The women on the pill reported drinking significantly less than the other women in the month preceding the testing. Maybe, Dr. Jones speculates, the decrease in drinking in both animals and women is related to slower ethanol metabolism. The effect of a drink lasts longer, so less alcohol is necessary. This leads to the possibility—still remote—that estrogens may provide protection against alcoholism. A tantalizing hint of this showed up when he noticed that women taking female hormones after hysterectomies tended to metabolize the alcohol more slowly and lower their alcohol intake. If they stopped the medication, they started drinking again. He found a good number of alcoholic women past menopause who were not on hormones and who drank heavily. In a look at the future, which may bring more understanding of this significant interrelationship, Dr. Jones suggests, "Estrogen therapy with alcoholic women may be particularly helpful with women who have experienced gynecological problems or severe depression that resulted in lowered sex hormonal levels. We would like to point out that to our knowledge there is no experimental data to support our contention." There is also the unanswered question of how the risk of cancer from prolonged use of estrogens should be weighed against the risks of alcoholism. Would the cure be worse than the disease?

There is conflicting evidence about alcohol use and abuse and gynecological problems. Some alcoholic women report starting their drinking bouts just before their periods begin, at the time they suffer from premenstrual tension. Others see no connection between the two events. When Dr. Jane E. James took a first look at women AA members for the Kansas City Area Council on Alcoholism, she found that fifty-four of the eighty-nine who answered her questionnaire said they drank more heavily just before or during their menstrual periods; of these, twenty-eight drank most before, fifteen during. This is also the time for the folk remedy of a good stiff drink to relieve menstrual cramps. Maybe, researchers speculate, as sex-hormone levels of estrogen and progesterone rise to a peak and suddenly fall, triggering menstruation, alcohol's sedative effects are particularly noticeable. The self-medication works and may lead to more drinking.

Alcohol can certainly disturb the menstrual cycle, which is dismayingly vulnerable to everything from strenuous exercise to anxiety to the common cold. In alcoholic women, menstruation sometimes ceases altogether as its delicate balance is disrupted by malnutrition as well as the drug. "This may be nature's way of protecting women from pregnancy," Dr. Sheila Blume, former medical director of the National Council on Alcoholism, suggests. "Many times, when a woman drinks heavily, her periods stop. I wouldn't worry about menstrual irregularity for six months after sobriety. Sometimes excessive vaginal bleeding begins with withdrawal from alcohol but we can treat it with hormones. Given time, the cycle reestablishes itself."

There is some evidence that other gynecological problems are associated with alcoholism. It isn't clear whether excessive drinking caused the trouble, or whether women who aren't sure of their femininity and also have sex-related physical problems are more likely to drink heavily. In one study Dr. Sharon Wilsnack, then at Harvard, found startling differences between alcoholic women and a control group of social drinkers, and the difficulties started before the drinking became a problem.[5] Over 25 percent of the married alcoholics said they had been unable to have children even though they had tried; only 4 percent of the other married women were involuntarily childless. More than three-quarters of the alcoholic women had had obstetrical or gynecological difficulties compared to 35 percent of the controls. These included sterility, repeated miscarriages, and trouble conceiving. Whether hormonal imbalances might have predisposed these women to gynecological problems—and also to alcoholism—is still a question. What is becoming clear is that alcohol affects the reproductive organs of women as well as those of men. Researchers at the University of Helsinki in Finland reviewed animal studies on this question in the scientific literature and found that female sex glands are harmed by chronic abusive drinking. This kind of damage shows up in sterility because of atrophied ovaries, menstrual irregularities, and decreased female sexual characteristics.[6] (See chapter 9, "Alcohol and Pregnancy.")

With increasing age, the rate at which alcohol leaves the body slows down and the effects of one drink may last longer. Women are especially vulnerable to another effect of the drug—its interference with the absorption of calcium. After menopause, the bent back and weak bones of osteoporosis handicap many women. If they also drink heavily, they cut down still more on the strength of their bones and make themselves even more vulnerable to falls and fractures. When Dr. Paul D. Saville checked the autopsy reports of sudden deaths in Manhattan, he found that bone density decreased noticeably in women over fifty; among alcoholic women, all under forty-five, he found bone densities like those of women over seventy.

Women also seem to be more prone to liver damage and pneumonia if they drink excessively. A study by Canada's Addiction Research Foundation showed that deaths from pneumonia are three times more prevalent among alcoholic men than in the general population; but in alcoholic women the figure reaches a fearful sevenfold increase.[7] The pneumonia deaths, of course, may just be a reflection of the fact that alcohol interferes with resistance to infectious disease, and women alcoholics are more likely to be hidden until they are terribly sick. The liver damage is more puzzling and may, perhaps, be tied in with the whole mystery of hormonal influences on a wide variety of body processes. London's *Daily Mirror* of June 10, 1977, reported that doctors at King's Hospital Liver Unit in London found a "significantly higher" incidence of alcoholic liver disease in women there, and were startled that it often occurred in those under forty-five. Men, by contrast, develop cirrhosis in their fifth or sixth decade.

On a more frivolous note, an English professor of microbiology points out what may be an advantage for women who use alcohol. Because their bodies produce their own alcohol, they may be able to challenge the results of urine tests for alcohol levels and might win acquittal on drunk-driving charges. Yeast, a common vaginal inhabitant, will produce alcohol from sugar in the blood and may contaminate the urine sample, making it impossible to tell whether the driver had been drinking or just had an infection.

On the whole, though, the particular physical problems women face when they abuse alcohol lead to the unpleasant possibility that alcohol may be more dangerous for women than for men. As with most other drugs, physical damage results when there are repeated large doses—the occasional drinker does no harm to her body and may even do some good. Subtle intellectual functioning however, seems vulnerable even to small amounts of this potent substance. Most people would agree, though, that minor memory lapses are a small price to pay for the relaxation that a few drinks can bring. As a matter of fact, dulling the rational animal is a major reason for social drinking. As William James observed in his classic *The Varieties of Religious Experience,* "The sway of alcohol over mankind is unquestionably due to its power to stimulate the mystical faculties in human nature, usually crushed to earth by the cold facts and dry criticism of the sober hour. Sobriety diminishes, discriminates and says no. Drunkenness expands, unites and says yes."

It also causes problems, and it is clear that certain realities of women's lives expose them to increased hazards when alcohol is abused. In a small pilot study the Metropolitan Life Insurance Company found that 20 percent of the home accidents in which women died involved alcohol. And at Peter Bent Brigham Hospital in Boston doctors noticed that alcohol (which dulls judgment) and smoking (which provides the flame) were, when combined, the most prominent factors in causing severe burns. More than 80 percent of the women who are heavy drinkers are also smokers. Dr. Francis D. Moore, one of the internationally recognized surgeons who conducted the study, commented, "There are plenty of burn-prone men but the older middle-aged woman who gets burned after drinking and smoking represents a recurrent theme." Women were more likely than men to be victims, usually igniting their hair or clothing. The problem is nationwide. A middle-aged divorcée was comfortably watching television in her Los Angeles apartment, wearing only a nightgown, when she put her drink down and lit a cigarette. "The nightgown just exploded," she told the doctor who treated her for extensive burns on her face, neck, and arms.

Since women are more likely to go to doctors' offices than men—and doctors prescribe more psychoactive drugs for women—they are at high risk of stumbling into trouble. The pills they pop into their mouths, combined with alcohol, can lead to side effects that range from annoying headaches to irreversible coma and death. Betty Ford, the former First Lady, fought what her son called "a very, very rough battle against the effects of Valium and alcohol." Mrs. Ford suffers from a painful arthritic condition. Her son Steve said the problem probably arose because of "too many doctors giving medication." Mrs. Ford herself courageously announced she was struggling with alcoholism as well as dependence on other drugs—a classic double addiction. Many doctors don't bother to ask questions or warn their patients of possible interactions. Dr. Blume, who teaches medical students, says, "A lot of what doctors know or think they know is cultural knowledge of alcohol. They haven't been taught much. The new generation of medical students is going to be alert to the dangers of prescribing certain drugs without warning about alcohol use. In previous years, no one ever thought about it."

Dr. Blume credits the Karen Ann Quinlan case, which brought international attention to the difficulties in determining when death occurs, with changing the medical climate. The young woman went into an irreversible coma reportedly because she combined alcohol and Valium, the most widely used and abused prescription drug.

Doctors have been programmed by medical advertising to prescribe in a manner that Dr. LeClair Bissell of New York describes as "sexist." The ads indicate, she says, that "a man needs a tranquilizer because he has had a heart attack. A woman needs one because she's harried, uneasy, or the bridge club has been critical. Men get tranquilizers for medical, physical reasons. Women get them to get them out of the office."

This picture of woman as more vulnerable has a long, respectable history. Aristotle saw her as "more compassionate than Man, more ready to weep, but at the same time more jealous, more querulous, more inclined to abuse. In addition she is an easy prey to despair and less sanguine than Man, more shameless and less jealous of honor, more untruthful, more easily disappointed, and has a longer memory."

As usual women themselves have adopted this view and, although it doesn't absolve doctors and pharmaceutical manufacturers from responsibility, women themselves are in part responsible for overprescription. Dr. Robert L. DuPont, former head of the National Institute on Drug Abuse in Washington, says, "There is, in fact, no evidence that physicians more often prescribe psychoactive drugs for women patients with psychological symptoms than they do for men with similar symptoms. Women do, however, typically report higher levels of psychic symptoms than do men. And it is, of course, more permissible in our society for women and particularly older women to admit to psychic distress and to seek medical aid for it. With changing sex-role expectations, we anticipate that members of both sexes will feel freer to admit to psychic pain and to seek help for it."

A doctor whose job it is to relieve suffering feels impelled to do something. If he can't do anything else, handing a piece of paper across a desk is a symbolic gesture, and sleeping pills and tranquilizers are among the most common drugs prescribed (even though there is now doubt that sleeping pills work when used for more than two consecutive weeks). Adding alcohol to these drugs is like adding a downer to a downer, and the results can be fatal. Alcohol and barbiturates, in particular, show a synergistic effect—put the two together, and the result is more than you'd expect just by adding equivalent doses. One estimate, based on the usual mythical 150-pound man with an empty stomach, is that it may take twelve or thirteen quick drinks in succession to push the blood-alcohol level high enough to cause death; but as little as two or three drinks in a short time combined with the usual dose of one or two barbiturate tablets at bedtime has been fatal. This may explain some of the "accidental suicides" of famous show-business personalities such as Dorothy Kilgallen and Judy Garland. A few sleeping pills after a few drinks, and they never woke up.

Some antidepressants, when used with alcohol, which is itself a depressant, can also dangerously retard the central nervous system. And the common painkiller Darvon is also tricky to use if alcohol is in the picture because it increases the intoxicating effects of drinking. A drug that is given chiefly to women and their sexual partners, Flagyl—which treats vaginal infections caused by a fungus—sometimes interacts with alcohol to produce headache and nausea, reason enough to avoid drinking while taking it.

One of the most devastating interactions occurs with antidepressants known as monoamine oxidose (MAO) inhibitors (Marplan or Parnate, for example), often prescribed for postmenopausal depression. A woman who innocently drinks certain kinds of chianti while on these pills can be thrown into an "acute hypertensive crisis" (extremely high blood pressure)—a stroke, heart attack, and even blindness can result.

For the alcoholic woman, there are special problems. Even

when she has been "dry" for years, certain drugs—warfarin, dilantin, tolbutamide, and isoniazid among them—are only half as effective in her body. She may need twice as much as someone else for the drug to do its work. Also, someone who has developed a tolerance to alcohol, although there is none in her system at the moment, will need larger than usual doses of barbiturates or anesthesia. This is important in surgery, where the amount commonly used will not put the patient into a deep, painfree sleep. On the other hand, if a woman has been drinking she will need less of these drugs to produce the same effect and should be honest about her drinking history to avoid an overdose.

Since alcohol diffuses so easily throughout the body and affects all body systems, it's not surprising that combining it with other drugs produces unpleasant and sometimes dangerous side effects. But people are not test tubes, and their reactions when drugs are mixed in them are not always predictable. One person may react violently to a drug combination that won't disturb another at all. What's important is that the patient realize that adding alcohol to another drug will probably result in an effect that is different from using either one or the other alone.

The accompanying chart lists some of the drugs most widely used by women and what to watch out for if they are taken by someone who drinks. In view of the number of possible reactions, Dr. Frank Seixas, a former medical director of the National Council on Alcoholism, warns, "For many moderate drinkers, the knowledge that so many important drug interactions exist may suggest to the physician to advise caution in all drinking whenever other drugs have been prescribed."

Women—who use more over-the-counter and prescription drugs than men—have a special obligation to understand what happens when they use the world's oldest tranquilizer—alcohol— with today's array of wonder drugs.

DRUG INTERACTIONS WITH ALCOHOL

Chemical or Generic Name	Common or Brand Name	Use	Possible Effects
Digitalis	Digoxin, Digitoxin	Heart stimulant	Increased effect on heart; arrhythmias
Nitroglycerin		Treatment of angina	Increased effect on heart
Amitriptyline and others	Elavil, Norpramin, Tofranil, Vivactil	Antidepressant	Increased sedative effect; coma; increased effect of alcohol
Warfarin	Coumadin	Anticoagulant	Long-standing, heavy alcohol use may lead to faster rate of metabolism
Phenytoin sodium	Dilantin	Antiepileptic	Long-standing, heavy alcohol use may lead to faster rate of metabolism
Phenylbutazone	Butazolidin	Treatment of arthritis	Long-standing, heavy alcohol use may lead to faster rate of metabolism
Antituberculous drugs	Isoniazid, Streptomycin	Treatment of tuberculosis	Long-standing, heavy alcohol use may lead to faster rate of metabolism and acute intoxication
Disulfiram	Antabuse	Deter drinking	Flushing; nausea; palpitations; shock
Tolbutamide and others	Orinase, Diabinese	Oral treatment of diabetes	Antabuse-like effect
Insulin		Treatment of diabetes	Fluctuates blood-sugar level
Metronidazole	Flagyl	Vaginal infection	Headache; nausea
Griseofulvin	Fulvicin	Skin fungus infection	Flushing; nausea
Furazolidone	Furoxone	Urinary tract infections	Antabuse-like effect
Aluminum-containing antacids	Maalox	Stomach distress	Depletes phosphorus—possibly fatal
Barbiturates	Amytal, Quaalude, Nembutal, Phenobarbital, Seconal	Sedative	Reduced driving skills; coma; death
Antihistamines	Benadryl, Chlor-Trimeton and others	Antiallergen	Reduced driving skills in small doses
Diazepam and others	Valium, Librium	Minor tranquilizers	Increased effect of alcohol; reduced driving skills

Drug	Brand	Type	Effect with alcohol
Glutethimide	Doriden	Sedative; deep sleep	Reduced driving skills
Chloral hydrate	Noctec	Sleep	Central nervous system depression; irregular heartbeat; flushing
Monoamine oxidase (MAO) inhibitors	Marplan, Parnate	Antidepressant	Drastic effects when combined with chianti; acute hypertensive crisis
Penicillin, Chloramphenicol	V-Cillin, Bicillin, Chloromycetin, etc.	Antibiotics	Interferes with absorption of antibiotic
Acetylsalicylic acid	Aspirin	Analgesic	Gastrointestinal bleeding
Acetaminophen	Tylenol, Datril	Analgesic	Gastrointestinal bleeding
Carisoprodol, Methocarbamol	Soma, Robaxin	Muscle relaxant	Enhanced depressant effect
Propoxyphene	Darvon	Analgesic	Depressed respiration; central nervous system depression after heavy alcohol ingestion
Lithium	Lithane, Eskalith	Antidepressant	Reduced driving skills
Ethchlorvynol	Placidyl	Sedative	Central nervous system depression
Meprobamate	Miltown	Minor tranquilizer	Reduced driving skills
Flurazepam	Dalmane	Sedative	Central nervous system depression; coma
Phenothiazine derivatives	Thorazine, Stelazine	Antipsychotic	Reduced driving skills
Haloperidol	Haldol	Antipsychotic	Reduced driving skills
Propanolol and others	Inderal, Aldomet, Catapres	Treatment of high blood pressure	Dangerously lowered blood pressure
Chlorothiazide and others	Diuril, Lasix	"Water pills" (diuretic)	Reduced blood pressure on standing; dizziness

Source: Based on information in Frank J. Ascione, "Caution: These Drugs Interact with Alcohol," *Pharmacy Times* (January 1978): 79–85 and Frank A. Seixas, "Alcohol and Its Drug Reactions," *Annals of Internal Medicine* 83 (July 1975): 86–92.

7

For Medicinal Purposes Only

*T*here is a charming, four-thousand-year-old Persian legend that a woman first discovered the health-giving properties of wine. Typically, her name has not survived, only the name of the man she served, King Jamshid. An Odysseuslike mythical figure, Jamshid loved to eat fresh grapes. After the harvest he ordered them stored in huge pottery vats in the cellar of his palace. Unfortunately, some of the grapes soured, and when he tasted the awful stuff he was convinced that the fruit had become poisonous. Like any good absolute monarch, he never knew when he might need a fresh supply of such a potent weapon to eliminate troublemakers, so he ordered the grapes and their liquid decanted into smaller jars and stored in his private apartments. It was there that the lady of his court found them. Suffering miserably from "sick headaches," she had decided to end her life. When she saw the jars labeled "poison" she sipped from one, then sipped some more. Gradually, life that had seemed so dismal seemed bright and full of promise. She was overcome with drowsiness and slept.

The next day she came back for more, and secretly she finished all the liquid. When the king discovered that his supply had disappeared, he confronted the lady, and she confessed, telling him that the jars had not contained poison, but some magic elixir with marvelous powers to ease pain and generate joy. Being no fool, Jamshid deliberately let his grapes ferment from then on, and served the primitive wine to all the members of his court.

This story foreshadows the way women have used alcohol from ancient times to the present. The poison relieved Jamshid's lady's psychosomatic complaint; she drank in secret; since the potion was always available, she kept increasing her dosage; and when forced to by the man in her life, she admitted her guilty secret.

From the time of Jamshid onward (if you believe in legends), ethyl alcohol has been used as an anesthetic, a pain killer, as a way to lift the spirits of the dejected, and as a treatment for almost every ailment that assails mankind. It was the aspirin of the ancients. Dr. Salvatore Lucia, who has made an exhaustive study of wine's history, calls it "the oldest of medicines."

Noah has the dubious distinction of being the first recorded drunk, but by the time of Christ, the medicinal attributes of wine had become as well known as the intoxicating ones. St. Paul's prescription for Timothy was, "No longer drink only water, but use a little wine for the sake of your stomach and your frequent ailments."

By the Middle Ages, monks and doctors had concocted dozens of infusions of wine and herbs, with specific instructions for their use. Undaunted by reality, they claimed to cure everything from gout to sterility. In the most venerable printed collection of tested recipes for the aid of the ailing, Arnaldus of Villanova wrote that raisin wine "is proper for sick old people, also for melancholics and phlegmatics, and it particularly makes women fat." Ginger and cinnamon bark in wine was suggested "to beautify women . . . [and give] a white, subtle and pleasant complexion." Incidentally, it also cured paralysis. Rosemary wine had special importance "for it rectifies the uterus in the body and helps in childbirth." Modern Canadian doctors used alcohol to ease the pangs of labor. The treatment was brought home from World War II battlefields by surgeons who noticed alcohol's analgesic effects on wounded soldiers—another rediscovery of ancient wisdom.

Arnaldus, born in thirteenth-century Catalonia and heir to centuries of Arab domination, knew of an even more effective wine product. An Arab alchemist named Geber was reputed to have discovered about A.D. 800 the secret of heating the wine, then condensing the steam into something now known as brandy. The name he used was *alkuhl*, the word for the dark eyeliner of ground antimony still used by Eastern women. Gradually it came to mean any fine powder and then an essence. Eventually, it was adopted as the name for the essence of wine.

This potent product of distillation was neglected until Arnaldus touted its qualities as an *aqua vitae*—a "water of life." His claims for it sound like the come-ons of medicine-show barkers a few centuries later: "It prolongs life, clears away ill-humors, revives the heart and maintains youth," he exulted. Although Arnaldus's claims sound extravagant, a look at six thousand Californians showed that moderate drinkers really did live longer than abstainers or heavy drinkers. Researcher Nancy Day of the University of California at Berkeley has since found that lower death rates and moderate alcohol use go together presumably because alcohol increases the "good" cholesterol in the bloodstream.

In the fifteenth century, German doctor and surgeon Hieronymus Brunschwig suggested that a few spoonfuls of this powerful elixir each day would not only prolong life, but would cure deafness, end toothache, aid digestion, and heal wounds. Even his prescriptions were not too far-fetched. A stiff drink has been an age-old remedy for the pain of a raging tooth; alcohol and peppermint are a classic combination for calming an upset stomach; and from the time of the Greeks until Lister introduced carbolic acid in the nineteenth century, wine and its products were used to sterilize wounds.

Curiously enough, modern studies have shown that it is not the alcohol but another substance (possibly tannin) in the grape that inhibits the growth of bacteria. Even though the New Testament tells of the Good Samaritan pouring oil and wine into a traveler's wounds to heal him, the time-honored remedy fell into disrepute in the Middle Ages. The theory then was that pus was a curative substance, and soldiers treated by eminent professors of medicine were subjected to the torture of having metal prods inserted into their wounds so festering would take place. As a result they died agonizing deaths in great numbers. A few conservatives like Ambroise Paré of France followed the compelling evidence of their observations. They poured wine into the wounds, brought the edges together, and watched their patients recover.

Wine kills other bacteria, too. A young soldier in the Mediterranean theater of operations during World War II noticed that although his companions were laid low by stomach upsets, the native population seemed buoyantly healthy. No fools, they followed the local custom of splashing a generous quantity of wine into their water. When he did this, his stomach settled down, too. Back in the States, tests showed that newly fermented red wine, in particular, kills bacteria that cause diarrhea.

More recently two Canadian virologists, Dr. Jack Konowalchuk and Mrs. Joan I. Spiers, have reported that red wine kills the viruses that cause polio, cold sores, and some gastrointestinal illnesses—in the test tube, at least.[1] As evidence that it isn't the alcohol but tannin in the grapes that acts as a "magic bullet," they found that unfermented grape juice was an even more efficient antiseptic.

With or without scientific confirmation, doctors from the sixteenth through the nineteenth centuries prescribed wine for a bewildering variety of reasons. Sherry-sack was even recommended to ward off plague during the disastrous 1665 London epidemic. The use of the panacea had, by this time, become more refined. Specific types of wine were recommended for specific situations. The well-stocked medicinal wine cellar included champagne to prevent or ameliorate seasickness and less fashionable types of nausea; port for the treatment of fevers and anemia (possibly because its dark color resembled blood); white wine as diuretics; port, sherry, and Madeira to infuse strength into the invalid; and claret and burgundy to stimulate the appetite.

An ancient mixture recommended by Paracelsus in the sixteenth century continued to be used through the nineteenth and even into the twentieth. This Zurich-born physician and alchemist developed *vinum ferri*, a combination of wine (three glasses of which, we now know, provides 25 percent of daily iron requirements) and iron itself as a treatment for anemia. Iron filings were allowed to rust in wine, and then the fortified liquid was drained off. This unappetizing but effective combination was one of the early ancestors of the tonics that crowded the shelves of pharmacies during the 1800s, the golden age of patent medicines. The tonics and the even more potent bitters of that era promised to revive weak blood and make every woman her own medical expert.

It's not that doctors didn't have remedies to prescribe; it's just that the professionals were hard to get to and not too highly respected. A trip to fetch a doctor might mean an hour or two of bumpy riding on a horse or in a carriage, and was not to be considered for minor ailments. Besides, there was often a lack of confidence in the doctor's professional ability and in the efficacy of whatever the physician did suggest. One observer of the medical scene as late as 1870 noted that even prestigious Harvard Medical School didn't require written exams because so many of the students could not write well enough for such tests to be fair.[2]

It was a lot easier (and often safer) to go into the general store or pharmacy and, trusting to the claims on the label or local recommendations, pick a bottle that would do the trick. Never at a loss for ingenuity or extravagant claims, these ready-made medicines promised to prevent falling hair, build up the rundown, cure cancer, kidney diseases, and deafness and, most frequently, ameliorate those ubiquitous disorders known as "female complaints." Almost all the nostrums had a fortifying quantity of alcohol as a basic part of the formula.

The tonics usually had modest amounts, but some popular bitters had more alcohol than some whiskey. Oxygenated Bitters, made in Windsor, Vermont, for example, contained about 40 percent alcohol—80-proof by current standards. No wonder that Mary E. Hanover wrote in 1851 in glowing terms of how it had helped her overcome diarrhea, weakness, and spirits so low "I felt as if nothing could ever make me cheerful again." After buying a supply she announced, "However surprising, it is nevertheless sure that I was almost immediately relieved of every symptom of my various complaints, and gained so rapidly that I was a wonder to all who knew me after using four or five bottles of the medicine." Mrs. Hanover was a true descendant of King Jamshid's lady. The recommended dosage was one tablespoonful three times a day on an empty stomach. Even men and women who had signed the temperance pledge could allow themselves a strengthening dose now and then "for medicinal purposes only." On an empty stomach, it was far more effective than the forbidden beer could ever have been.

But this was just the beginning of the age of self-medication. The real peak came with the development and merchandising of Lydia E. Pinkham's Vegetable Compound, the most successful patent medicine ever sold. (It is still on drugstore shelves today.) Mrs. Pinkham first made her concoction in the family kitchen with her three sons and a daughter helping to fill the bottles. She gave them away out of the kindness of her heart to suffering females for whom she acted as a neighborhood Florence Nightingale. According to one version of her rags-to-riches saga, the formula, never a secret, came to her through her husband, who took it in exchange for twenty-five dollars owed him by a local Lynn, Massachusetts, mechanic. This herbal cure "for the weakness of females" contained pleurisy root, black cohosh, and fenugreek seed—and 18 percent alcohol "solely as a solvent and preservative" (wine contains 12–14 percent). An abolitionist, fighter for human rights, and staunch member of the Woman's Christian Temperance Union, Mrs. Pinkham contributed to the well-being—and alcohol consumption—of millions of nondrinkers.

Profit making entered the picture when the 1873 financial panic shook her husband's always precarious monetary situation. When some elegant Salem ladies drove up to her dilapidated door and offered welcome cash for the bottles of tonic they'd heard would rid them of their troubles, Mrs. Pinkham gladly accepted five dollars for half a dozen containers. Business became so brisk that manufacturing soon moved from the kitchen to the basement, and her sons took to the road to promote sales. In what can only be called a stroke of genius, son Daniel suggested that his mother's picture adorn each label. Rising from a neat, pleated fichu it soon became the most widely recognized face in the country.[3]

Advertising that called the compound "an invaluable medicine for Women, invented by a Suffering Woman" appeared along with the prim, motherly emblem in newspapers published in small towns as well as big cities. In one year, the company is reputed to have spent an unheard-of one million dollars on advertising. Those were the days when Mrs. Pinkham's picture was often the only woman's face a weekly newspaper had readily available, so she did double duty as Queen Victoria when a royal illustration was required.[4]

As sales increased, so did jokes. One favorite went like this:

Young Lady: Oh, I've smashed my bottle of Lydia Pinkham's.

Mother: Aha, a compound fracture.

Men, too, got into the act. Irreverent Dartmouth students walked along campus paths chanting:

There's a face that haunts me ever,
There are eyes mine always meet;
As I read the morning paper,
As I walk the crowded street. . . .

The sight of the reassuring face was only one gimmick for increasing sales. Along with the detailed label which suggested the
compound's use "for prolapsus uteri or falling of the womb and
other female weaknesses . . . [and] for weakness of the generative
organs" (commonly condensed to "a baby in every bottle"), the
promoters of the tonic invited letters from troubled females, all to
be answered by Lydia Pinkham herself. For eight years she acted
as a combination Ann Landers and home medical adviser; after
her death in 1883, and despite announcements in major newspapers, the letters kept coming. They were answered as before by a
team of secretaries who had been trained in the proper approach.

Some of the letters made superlative advertising copy: "I would
have been in my grave ten years ago but for it. My womb had
fallen and rested on the bladder. The doctor could not relieve me;
my mind was deranged. Your Compound cured me. It helped me
through the change of life all right [even today, alcohol is an informal treatment for this inevitable female complaint]; am now in
good health. It has also cured my husband of kidney trouble; made
him like a new man. Please state my words in the strongest terms.
I am glad to send you my picture. I traveled twelve miles to have
it taken for you.—Mrs. W. L. Day, Bettsville, Ohio."

The letters sent in reply started "Dear Friend" and were concluded by "Yours for health." Deeply concerned about the igno-
rance many of her letter writers revealed, Mrs. Pinkham wrote
and distributed free a pioneering four-page pamphlet explaining
puberty, conception, childbirth, and menopause. In an age of
whispers and circumlocutions when a leg was a "limb," her language was precise and her physiology explicit and correct.

After twenty years, the compound was still selling for a dollar a
bottle (five dollars for six) and was purported to cure everything
from menstrual cramps to cancer. The company became the most
successful company ever to have been founded by a woman.

Theodore Roosevelt slowed the patent-medicine boom slightly
on June 30, 1906, when he signed the Pure Food and Drug Act, an
earnest but generally ineffective attempt to regulate self-medica-

tion. The law required that a list of dangerous or addictive ingredients be listed on labels, and banned "false and misleading advertising." It didn't ban the use of addictive agents, however, so soothing syrups for children still contained opium, Lydia Pinkham's still had an alcohol base, and coca beef tonic with sherry wine still contained cocaine. No prescriptions were necessary for these powerful mood changers. The modest spoonful of the suggested dosage was temptingly easy to exceed, and many people found themselves innocently hooked on one or another of these medicine-chest remedies. Women, prone to disorders that could only be hinted at, were particularly vulnerable to remedies kept within easy and private reach on the home shelf. And "female complaints" often yielded to the tranquilizing effects of alcohol, as King Jamshid's lady had discovered.

They also yielded to opium, as nineteenth-century doctors recognized. Between 1850 and 1920 (when the Harrison Act's regulation of narcotics went into full effect), twice as many women as men were addicted to opium. Among them was playwright Eugene O'Neill's mother, who had been given the drug to relieve pain following childbirth. At that time, alcoholism was seen as a man's disease and narcotic addiction as a woman's. Even now treatment centers report that women will readily admit to the use of drugs but deny their alcoholism. Patent medicines were often liberally laced with one or the other panacea, disguising addiction as treatment.[5]

One of the few generally recognized medical uses of alcohol was in the treatment of a "female complaint"—premature labor. The alcohol was administered intravenously, close to the end of pregnancy and, as in the following case, only if the course of the labor had not yet made delivery seem imminent.

At four-thirty one afternoon, a pregnant twenty-three-year-old was having a cup of coffee with her next-door neighbor when the cramps began. At first she felt what she thought was mild indigestion. Half an hour later the discomfort settled in the middle of her abdomen. Soon she realized that she was having mild contractions; she could feel her uterus tighten and harden, then relax. She was seven months pregnant. By five-thirty, she was damp with the fear that she would lose the baby. By eight-thirty, after a visit to her doctor's office to check that the contractions were really labor and that her cervix hadn't dilated yet, she was in the hospital. She was weighed, then put to bed. A 10 percent solution of alcohol, the amount calculated according to her weight, began dripping into her vein; rapidly at first, then more slowly. Twelve hours later the contractions had stopped completely. What she'd received in the way of alcohol was the equivalent of three stiff drinks of whiskey in two hours, an amount that would bring her blood-alcohol level up to 0.14. It was kept at about that level for twenty-four hours. (A blood-alcohol level of 0.1 is often the legal definition of intoxication, but an inexperienced drinker can feel very tipsy long before that.) The next day, on doctor's orders, she drank a screwdriver of vodka and orange juice every four hours, to maintain a moderate alcohol level. Once it seemed clear that the contractions weren't about to start again, temperance was reinstated. Two weeks later, with the time gained, she delivered a normal five-and-a-half-pound boy. There were no complications.

The remarkable ability of alcohol to calm uterine contractions was discovered in 1962 by reproductive biologist Anna Rita Fuchs while working with animals. She discussed her provocative results with her husband, Dr. Fritz Fuchs, later obstetrician and gynecologist in chief at the New York Hospital–Cornell Medical Center. He thought it might work on women, too. By a curious turn of fate, the first patient on whom he tried this new technique was his wife, who had gone into premature labor when she was seven months pregnant. Administered intravenously or by mouth, alcohol was used on more than 350 patients at the medical center and at hundreds of other hospitals in this country and abroad. Dr. Fuchs reported that two out of three cases were helped. "What probably happens," he explains, "is that alcohol interferes with the release of oxytocin by the pituitary gland. Oxytocin is the hormone that signals the body to begin labor. Patients given this treatment don't get drunk; that's something that happens in social situations. What usually happens is they just get drowsy and sleepy. There are no aftereffects on either the fetus or the mother."

Other obstetricians were less sanguine about the effects of the treatment on the mother, and new drugs plus knowledge about the harmful effects of high levels of alcohol on the fetus have made this treatment obsolete.

Every minute counts in two other medical uses of alcohol. If it can be infused (or guzzled) quickly enough, alcohol can save the lives of poison victims who have swallowed antifreeze (ethylene glycol) or formaldehyde. The victims are either curious children or adults attempting suicide. What happens is that the alcohol prevents the production of a poisonous by-product, and the antifreeze is quickly and harmlessly secreted. Formaldehyde becomes formic acid and also leaves the body safely.

Forty years ago, alcohol had many other widely approved uses. In the form of whiskey, brandy, or cordials it formed a basic part of official medical treatment to lower fevers, stimulate the heart, treat shock and frostbite, aid digestion and, of course, counteract snakebite. It was considered so indispensable that during Prohibition, doctors were allotted twenty-eight bottles of booze a year—for their patients, of course. Most of these uses have survived the onslaught of newer knowledge and remedies in a kind of underground layman's resistance to scientific advances. A nationwide survey in 1969 put "medical uses" third in a listing of good things that can be said about alcohol, right after "it helps people mix socially" and "helps people relax." It seems only common sense that alcohol makes you warmer if you're cold—doesn't a slug of whiskey bring a glow to the face and the stomach? The dismal truth is that alcohol dilates peripheral blood vessels—that's what makes a person seem warmer. Actually, this dilation encourages surface heat loss, so body temperature drops. What about the traditional hot toddy for a cold or the flu? Again, the liquor lowers body temperature when an even keel is what's helpful. The same effect destroys any benefit from alcohol used for shock and snakebite—it doesn't help either; it hurts, by lowering blood pressure. Pharmacologists Chauncy D. Leake and Milton Silverman, in their book *Alcoholic Beverages in Clinical Medicine,* regretfully advise: "If alcohol in any form is to be administered in the event of snakebite, it should be given to the bystanders." The sad reality is that most of the tried and true medicinal uses turn out to be based on myth and do more harm than good. So much for common sense.

What, then, is left? Dr. Morris Chafetz, the maverick of the alcohol establishment, thinks there are still a number of ways alcohol can be helpful. It can, he says, relax clogged nasal passages and make the cold sufferer more comfortable. It calms the anxiety that makes the pain of angina pectoris so unbearable. In chronic illness, it can make life more pleasant although, of course, it cures nothing more than boredom.

Alcohol also has a respected history as "a balm for the autumnal years." Maimonides, the twelfth-century philosopher, said of wine, "Old people need it most." In the past decade there have been many studies showing that institutionalized older people are happier when they are allowed moderate use of alcoholic beverages—particularly when the drinking is done with other people. One pilot project conducted by Dr. Brian L. Mishare of Harvard Medical School set up social get-togethers five days a week for residents in two old-age homes who did not have a history of alcohol problems. A wide variety of liquor was available (most residents chose whiskey) at no charge. The socialization—plus the small amounts of alcohol—decreased worry, increased the ease of getting to sleep, and didn't result in alcoholism or any physical problems.

Even veterinarians are convinced of the beneficial effects of alcohol on the old. One animal specialist prescribed ten drops of cognac in a demitasse spoon of water plus half an aspirin tablet to ease the undiagnosed aches and pains of a thirteen-year-old dog.

Dr. Salvatore Lucia, in his book *A History of Wine as Therapy*, goes even further than the Harvard researchers. He reports on studies (particularly in Italy) that suggest wine has beneficial effects on the circulatory system, which seem to prevent heart attacks. (This may be a mixed blessing, though; alcohol also weakens the heart muscle so that heart attacks may be fewer, but congestive heart failure more likely. See chapter 3, "Effects on Body and Brain.") He also credits the beverage with lowering the cholesterol level in the blood, a finding confirmed by several large-scale studies. As for diabetics who are usually denied alcohol on their highly restrictive diets, Dr. Lucia cites experts who claim that dry white wine, at least, may be beneficial. Wine, he reports, may even play a part in preventing the development of diabetes by speeding up the metabolism of carbohydrates and thereby decreasing the blood-sugar level.

More recent research, though, casts doubt on some of these uses. Dr. Ernest Noble, once head of the NIAAA, has reviewed the latest findings and says remorselessly, "Alcohol affects carbohydrate metabolism in a very complex and bizarre fashion. . . . Although many borderline diabetics under diet control do not suffer undue consequences from small amounts of alcohol, in view of the potentially dangerous and unpredictable reactions, abstinence from alcohol would seem the wisest course."[6]

One of the medically respected uses of alcohol has long been to relieve the pain of angina pectoris. The theory was that alcohol dilates the blood vessels leading to the heart (as nitroglycerin does) and allows the blood to flow freely. Dr. Irving S. Wright, former president of the American Heart Association, has written, "Few if any drugs for dilating the arteries are as effective." Time and improved scientific tools, however, have refuted that statement, too. They show that the arteries leading to the heart are not affected by doses of liquor, although smaller blood vessels certainly are enlarged. What a drink actually does for the sufferer is act as a mild anesthetic; it may blunt the pain, but it doesn't improve the condition. Nitroglycerin is far more effective.

Also more effective are drugs to lower blood pressure (for which wine has been recommended in the past), reduce cholesterol, and do half a dozen other things for which alcohol has been favored. But there are still doctors who suggest it, particularly in Europe. There are even some in this country who point out that it is more acceptable to a lot of people and has fewer side effects than pills or shots. Its respected history, they say, shouldn't be discarded. Many experts in the field of alcoholism see this as dangerous nonsense.

Dr. Sheila B. Blume puts it this way: "I have seen alcoholic patients who started to drink because their doctor recommended a shot of brandy or Scotch to relax them at bedtime. I have seen others who routinely drank tea laced heavily with brandy for menstrual cramps (sometimes at their physician's suggestion). One woman with a colicky baby was told by her pediatrician the only help he could suggest was a glass of brandy—for her. You can't look at alcohol as a medication. If you do, you are taking it as a drug, and as a drug it's addicting, dangerous, and occasionally fatal, especially when coupled with other drugs."

Dr. Frank Seixas concurs: "I'm against the use of wine or liquor as medication," he says. "It's there, so the person will tend to use more and more, particularly if it is recommended by an authority for regular use. It's all right occasionally—as an appetite stimulant, for instance—but I wouldn't recommend it for someone who has a serious problem with eating. That puts it into the class of any other prescribed medication, and with alcohol nobody keeps an eye on the number of refills you get."

Even without the aura of medical authority, it is hard to manage as self-medication. Mary Ann, who lives in Madison, Wisconsin, told a newspaper reporter doing a story on alcoholics that she had had her first drink at thirty. That's when her husband ran off with her best friend. Following time-honored custom, she took a drink at night, "as a tranquilizer so I could get to sleep." Within six months, the glass a night had become a quart a day.

As for the current craze—wine and candlelight as sex therapy—Dr. Shirley Smoyak told the National Nurses Society on Alcoholism that she didn't see this as a good way to cure anxiety or impotence. "It gets a little unhandy if you need that all the time," she said.

What many experts seem to be saying is that alcohol shouldn't be used for medicinal purposes, except to neutralize certain poisons. Its dosage is difficult to control and it is, for ten people out of every one hundred who drink, an addicting drug. One AA member summed it up this way, "Because alcohol makes you feel good, you can easily learn to turn to it when you feel lousy." It is so troublesome to use that Dr. Robert B. Forney told an American Medical Association convention, "If it were just going on the market now, it would be available only by prescription."

8

Alcohol and the Family

*I*n its unsteady march through time, alcohol has been hailed as God's gift to mankind and as a demon that destroys home and health. The Jewish marriage ceremony begins with a cup of wine as a symbol of joy; righteous Temperance ladies vowed that "lips that touch liquor shall never touch mine." A New York City psychotherapist who has been a people-watcher for twenty-five years is convinced that "alcohol has saved more marriages than it's ended, prevented more beatings than it's caused. It softens the hard edges of life." Yet a Gallup poll reported by the *New York Times* (February 13, 1977) showed a 50 percent rise in the number of American families concerned about the damage alcohol was causing in their lives. (By 1982 one-third of those interviewed said alcohol had caused family problems.) And the federal government estimated in 1976 that thirty-six million Americans were caught in the web of alcohol abuse—victims of unhappy marriages, broken homes, desertion, divorce, poverty, and childhood neglect.[1]

Most drinkers, of course, are social drinkers, and no one has counted up the times families have been warmed and brought together by eggnog at Christmas or a nightcap to end a tense day. A drink at the end of a working day has often acted like the defusing of a grenade. It provides just enough calm to allow perspective to return and marks the division between a growling office personality and the ease of home.

The role of alcohol as a marriage saver has been observed by therapists puzzled about why certain people stay together despite problems that would blow other relationships apart. "If they're both in a haze, they can avoid looking at what's bothering them," is how one counselor put it. More bluntly, as Mercedes McCambridge said, "If Barbara gets a little bombed and Harry gets a little bombed they can go to sleep and not be forced to lie in connubial bliss for at least one more night. . . ."

On the other hand, whatever the physiological realities (see chapter 3, "Effects on Body and Brain"), some women say that a few drinks make them feel more receptive sexually. A family counselor at the Nassau County, New York, Department of Drug and Alcohol Addiction found: "There are women who drink so they can perform sexually. It lowers inhibitions. Women who live with an alcoholic can drink and let their hair down. When they're sober they pull back and can't perform, even though they're not alcoholic." Dr. Ben Morgan Jones, studying young moderate drinkers in Oklahoma, says many of his subjects have reported increased sexual feelings—throbbing and tingling in the vaginal area, a sensation of warmth—after one or two drinks, and speculates that fact is not far from folklore where sex and alcohol are concerned. Heavier drinking, though, may lead to disinterest in sex and even to a lack of sensation in the vaginal area. A schoolteacher, caught in an unhappy marriage, told her therapist she made a point of drinking a lot every night to avoid sex. "I was always dead asleep when my husband crawled into bed. Nothing could wake me."

Several studies show that sexual difficulties and dissatisfactions are typical of alcoholic marriages. So is divorce.[2] Alcoholic marriages have seven times as many separations and divorces as those in the general population.[3] But a woman alcoholic is more likely to be divorced than a man.[4] A woman will stay with a man who drinks too much because, as one counselor emphasizes, "It's still a man's world in terms of finances and economics. If women have a family and kids, they're not going to leave so quickly. For an alcoholic man, the last thing to go is the paycheck." Dr. Ruth Fox, a pioneer in treating alcoholism, has found that men "are more apt to pack up and leave an alcoholic wife whom they feel they can no longer love." Judy Fraser of Canada's Addiction Research Foundation estimated that nine out of ten men leave alcoholic wives, but nine out of ten women stay with their alcoholic husbands.

This is a shocking statistic, but one that seems to be only common sense. Like most statistics in this field, however, it has to be considered with care. The idea of men as the model against whom everything must be measured distorts the picture of the woman alcoholic. The reality is that there are more divorcées, whether they are alcoholic or not. Women marry earlier, live longer, and are less likely to remarry, so there are more single women around. Measuring women against women may show that alcoholic women don't differ much from other women in their rates of separation and divorce. There is already some evidence that alcoholic women aren't necessarily discarded.

In a study of white, mostly Protestant middle-class alcoholic women in the Philadelphia area, Drs. Howard P. Wood and Edward L. Duffy found that their marriages were "remarkably long lasting and free of infidelity." Other small studies of middle- and upper-class women have confirmed this finding. Then, of course, there are the populations—usually hospitalized or imprisoned lower-class women—who do seem to have higher divorce rates than men with similar problems. What this means is what the perceptive novelist and essayist Aldous Huxley cautioned about: "Generalizing about Woman is like indicting a Nation—an amusing pastime, but very unlikely to be productive of truth or utility." There is no typical Alcoholic Woman; the problems an alcoholic woman faces in life seem to be closely related to how many socioeconomic cushions she has to protect her from harsh reality. It is also possible that studies showing women more likely to be deserted are based on women in treatment; since this is only a small fraction of the alcoholic population—usually the one with the fewest resources—any attempt to generalize these findings to all women or to compare them to men (who are more likely to be treated earlier) has to be examined with a critical eye. Once the end of the line has been reached, marriages crumble for both men and women.

For a while, though, alcohol may have been the "enabling drug," providing missing feelings of adequacy and acceptability and meeting the needs of both partners, even if only one of them used it. Many women are encouraged by their husbands to drink.

"In each case," Drs. Wood and Duffy noticed, "alcohol at first seemed to release the drinker from her anxieties about herself, facilitating self-expression and making her feel she was the person she's always wanted to be." Later, alcohol released anger, "with a built-in eraser." How could an understanding husband hold her responsible? "I didn't know what I was doing. I was drunk."

There are many ways an alcoholic wife provides the emotional setting that keeps a marriage together. One loyal husband confided to his counselor that he liked his wife's rages. They kept him sexually excited: "We've been married twenty years and we have seven children. Why did I stay with her? For the sex."

There's also the man who was abused as a child and is sitting on a keg of rage himself. As one therapist says, "He needs an excuse to abuse a woman. If his wife drinks too much she gives him a perfect excuse. He has structured his life so he can hit." This man is the sort of person who needs a "bad guy" so he can feel like the "good guy." He has an investment in his wife's alcoholism. His self-esteem rises as hers goes down. She is "sick"—he is "well."

Even when there is no physical conflict, alcoholic marriages are often emotionally unrewarding. Drs. Wood and Duffy, whose study is one of the very few of alcoholic wives, found that they tended, in psychological terms, to marry their mothers! These middle-class woman had often grown up in homes where the alcoholic father was the nurturing one—warm, responsive. The mother, on the other hand, seemed cold and domineering, a perfectionist who could never be satisfied. The men the daughters married were often domineering and emotionally distant, too. When the husbands were unable to give or receive love, the wives, like their fathers, turned to alcohol. Surprisingly, these marriages endured, perhaps because both husband and wife needed emotional distance to stay together. When she was drunk she was, in effect, no longer there, no longer making emotional demands he was not able to meet.

The woman who drinks too much may show striking similarities to the woman who marries an alcoholic and may or may not become a problem drinker herself. Both tend to come from families in which a parent (usually the father) was alcoholic. Often their early lives were disrupted by death or desertion. They both think little of themselves. As a family counselor has noticed, "A woman who lives with an alcoholic—like the woman alcoholic herself—

has terrible problems with self-esteem. She tells herself, 'If I were a better person he wouldn't drink.' They have the same economic problems. When a woman alcoholic is sober she has to compete in the job market, just like one who leaves an alcoholic husband. Both have to learn to trust other women."

In one way or another, they both try to repeat their own early family lives, no matter how much they may have suffered. "When I was a kid," a tense, lean, middle-aged woman told her therapist, "I swore I would never drink. I even refused to date guys who drank. Now, here I am, trying to get my husband to stop drinking, and maybe drinking too much myself. What went wrong?" It seems likely that a woman like this admired her mother, who seemed strong and invulnerable, keeping the family together and acting as both mother and father in an alcoholic home. She married an alcoholic to feel indispensable and like her mother. But she can't quite live up to her own ideal and needs to keep him in trouble so she can continue to feel superior. The woman who becomes alcoholic herself may have felt closer to her father; like him, she uses alcohol to solve her emotional problems in marriage.

The husbands of alcoholic wives go through a whole gamut of emotions and responses as the illness progresses. First comes denial: "My husband was out of town a lot. He didn't see anything. He didn't want to see anything. Friends finally got him to notice that I was sleeping an awful lot. Sometimes I would go to bed during my own dinner parties." Another husband finally faced the fact that his wife had a problem with alcohol when he realized how often she'd been hospitalized during the past few years. It was never for alcoholism, but there was the time she slipped and broke her wrist, the pneumonia, the intestinal bleeding.

Once the realization has come, there is an attempt to assign blame. Jacqueline P. Wiseman, professor of sociology at the University of California in San Diego, found that the blaming took different forms when the woman was alcoholic. Wives often feel at fault if their husbands drink too much—"I've failed as a wife, I've failed in my marriage." Husbands don't worry about how they might have failed; the blame is obviously with the drinking wife. And, true to the culture pattern which decrees that women support the opinions of their men, the wives agree.

When a woman confronts her drinking husband, he often counters with: "It's your nagging that drives me to it. If only you were different, I wouldn't drink." The alcoholic woman also places at least part of the blame on her spouse, but her complaint is a different one. "You've left me alone all the time with the children. I feel deserted." Loneliness is a recurring theme. Even in their complaints, they are bound by their sex-roles, reflecting their different situations in the marriage.

The emphasis may shift from blame to protection. For one thing, there is the need to hide the special horror a woman drunk produces. "My father wouldn't get anyone in to take care of us kids," one girls remembers, "because he was afraid people would find out my mother drank." Then there is the wish that, given love and time, this too shall pass away. A suburban woman recalls, "I was a strange kind of mother because I didn't know what it was like to be in a car pool. My husband took away the keys." Sometimes the protection takes the form of supplying liquor, so the woman won't have to go out to buy it. "He felt the streets were dangerous," a city woman says, "so he would leave me enough to drink each morning before he went to work. He was protecting me from getting mugged if I went to the store."

In kindness, too, husbands may decide to "do something" to end the drinking. One man set his wife up in business to keep her occupied, so she wouldn't drink. Another took the family on a long camping trip, away from the temptations of civilization. This is what AA members call "the environmental cure." It is just one more way of avoiding coming to grips with the problem.

Another technique used by both men and women is "Let's Pretend." "Maybe, if we all act as if nothing is wrong, the drinking will quietly go away." The husband tries not to nag or complain; plans are made as if they could be carried out; the children are kept in the dark. The whole family lives a delusion. One woman, whose husband had left her, continued to act as if they were still together. She wore her wedding ring. She included him in her everyday conversation, reporting what he did or said. If a friend pressed her for information, she developed a pounding headache and took to her bed. Only prolonged treatment helped her live with reality instead of fantasy.

All these ploys build up frustration and finally, rage. "I wash my hands of her," is the exasperated attitude. At one private sanatorium on Long Island, workers have noticed that women—often professionals—come in by themselves or with the help of a friend.

Even former first lady Betty Ford entered a treatment center
without her husband; he was out of town mending political fences.
Men are accompanied by anxious wives bringing bathrobes and
slippers and asking about visiting hours. "Particularly if she's been
here before," one nurse says, "we won't hear from a woman's family for days. We usually call after three days, and even then it's
hard to get some husbands to show up." Sometimes, though, a
husband does stick by his alcoholic wife, "and then they're even
better than the wives of alcoholics about coming to treatment sessions and trying to do everything they can."

The marriage is also eaten away by lack of trust. "Alcoholics are
very clever," says one psychiatrist. "They learn to hide, to maneu-
ver. It takes a lot of intelligence to maintain alcoholism in a marriage." After her husband had discovered every other hiding place,
a housewife found what she thought was the ultimate receptacle,
her steam iron. Another woman—a writer who did a lot of business traveling—found she could hide liquor miniatures (the kind
served on airplanes) in the shoes on her closet shelf and always
have a supply on hand. She did another thing some alcoholic
women find necessary to keep the budget balanced. "I'm no way a
thief," she says, "but for about three years I stole butter and bacon
and meat so that I could use the money for liquor." The sneaking
and lying understandably make everything suspect. "Many men
accuse their wives of sexual infidelity," a counselor says. "They
don't believe anything they say."

If alcohol affects a marriage, it also affects the children of that
marriage. "Alcoholism isn't a spectator sport. Eventually the
whole family gets to play," Joyce Rebeta-Burditt wrote in her
perceptive novel, *The Cracker Factory*. More than six million
American children live in alcoholic homes.

Very young children are peculiarly vulnerable to the games alcoholic women play. When she adopted a baby, Carrie was convinced all her problems would end. "Yet even after I got him," she
confesses, "I kept on drinking. There was never a day when I went
without a drink. I would put him in his crib and then run out to
the liquor store. Several times my husband would find me passed
out cold and the baby crying in his crib." Single-parent families—
in 1984 there were more than nine million of them headed by
women—present special difficulties. A single mother's drinking
may be known only to her small children. Economically and emo-

tionally drained, she may drink too much and expect too much of her only companions. One divorced mother beat her eighteen-month-old child with an electric cord because she was making too much noise: "I had this awful headache and she just kept crying and crying. She should have kept quiet. She should have known better."

Toddlers with an inattentive drinking mother also get into more accidents and miss meals. In another example of documenting the obvious, Dr. Sharon Landesman-Dwyer of the University of Washington found that mothers who were moderate social drinkers gave their toddlers as much attention as women who didn't drink. While there was no data in this study on heavy drinkers, a surprising finding was that mothers who were heavy smokers tended to be restrictive and punishing.

With an alcoholic mother, neglect is the norm. "Sometimes it's physical, sometimes emotional," a family counselor says. "It's hard to tell which is worse. Having a mother who's there but not really available may be rougher than having one who hits you." Joy Baker, wife of the former Senate majority leader, remembers her own drinking bouts and the effect on her family. "I knew I was ruining the life of a lot of people," she says. "Number one, my husband, because he was at the end of his strength about what to do about me. And my kids were on their own—they couldn't come and say 'Look Mom, I have a problem,' because Mom had a bigger problem than they did. . . . They were all very close, but I was kind of an outsider."

Alcohol and family violence go together, and the child in an alcoholic family may be exposed to crushing experiences, emotionally and physically. Over 90 percent of the cases of child abuse and neglect seen in Canada's Northwest Territories in the 1970s involved alcohol. Some experts say that alcoholic women are more likely to abuse their children than alcoholic men—because they are with them more. No one denies that alcohol and child abuse and neglect are disturbingly frequent companions, as are alcohol and adult conflicts.

Children who grew up to abuse alcohol have also often been in the house when fights erupted between their parents. One estimate is that one or both had been drinking in 90 percent of the cases of wife abuse seen in a Milwaukee crisis center. "These figures aren't released," says Mark Goff, an evaluator of programs for alcoholics, "because people are afraid the reaction will be 'she asked for it.' There's no abuse if they've both been drinking. They're both at fault." In rape, too, he continues, "there's often alcohol involved on both sides. The attitudes people have towards rape and towards alcoholism are similar . . . 'They bring it on themselves.' Actually, exposure to this kind of violence may bring it on in their children."

Older children may find themselves playing roles they would never have fallen into if their mother had not been drinking. Typically, an older girl will take the place of her unavailable mother. She will care for younger children, cook dinner, and even be the one who listens to her father's problems at the end of a working day. This forced growing up can be tricky. One counselor estimates that half the women she sees at a treatment center for alcoholics and drug addicts were involved in incest with either a father or a brother. Most of them had alcoholic fathers; those with alcoholic mothers were often helpless replacements in bed as well as in the kitchen.

An older boy may play out his fantasies of being his mother's rescuer. When she drinks, he may protect her from her husband: "Don't you touch my mother, you animal." Often the fighting and unpleasantness permeate family life, putting children in parental roles and turning the adults into quarrelsome youngsters. "It's very strange," a counselor comments. "Children have a tendency to see the person who is drinking as ill, but they wonder what's the excuse for the one who's not drinking. They don't seem to realize that so much energy is involved in dealing with the illness that there's very little emotion left over for them."

When children have to grow up too fast, guilt, anger, and anxiety may be the emotional price. Often they do poorly in school, skip classes, withdraw, or get into fights. The particular tragedy of the family with an alcoholic mother is that the woman is usually so well hidden no one recognizes what lies behind the children's problems. But if the guilty secret comes out, the whole family may get help early. "You only hear about the awful things that happen to children," this counselor points out. "But sometimes they turn out to be stronger people because their mother's alcoholism got them into treatment before they were too damaged." Children have also been helped by Al-A-Teen, independent of AA but closely allied with it, which offers a chance for teen-agers to get together and talk over their problems. "You're not alone" and "It's not your fault" are major messages. Other family members are sometimes aided by Al-Anon, another independent AA offshoot that helps them detach themselves from the disruptive behavior of the alcoholic. "Now," a young father said, "if I come home and find the house a mess and dinner not cooked, I take the kids out and try to have a good time. I don't feel guilty about it. And I don't feel it's my job to do anything more than is absolutely necessary around the house. She has to work out her own problems." As grownups, the children of alcoholic parents now have their own Al-Anon-affiliated groups, where many find help for the first time.

But these self-help groups aren't for everyone. A high school student in a suburban town says, "It's bad enough having an alcoholic mother without admitting it to other people." There are few men in Al-Anon, perhaps because they find it hard to admit that they need outside help.

Children often feel isolated and like outsiders in the normal world. An art student in the obligatory jeans and shirt recalls, "It really used to bother me. I'd read those stories about Dick and Jane and Spot and I thought every other family in the world was like that. They all had breakfast together, and went ice skating and smiled a lot." Her family life was chaotic, with an alcoholic mother and a father who was a successful and eternally busy lawyer. As a teen-ager she became defiantly different; there was obviously no way she could be like Dick and Jane, so she cultivated her artistic tastes, wore secondhand long skirts and moth-eaten fur coats to school, and pretended to think parties were "the pits." She didn't bring friends home because she never knew what she would find.

One of the hardest things she had to cope with was that she couldn't count on anything. One day her mother might be warm and loving; the next, completely withdrawn. "Other kids knew what they were going to do over vacations. All I could be sure of was that whatever promises were made would be broken." Then there was the strain of living with her parents' guilt. "When my mother was sober," she says, "she'd try to make up to us for all the times she'd been drunk. One Christmas we wouldn't get any presents; the next we'd get embarrassingly elaborate things like a six-foot stuffed giraffe or a whole set of matching luggage."

Children whose sense of self has been fragmented by the capricious giving and taking away of love in an alcoholic family are disturbingly likely to marry alcoholics themselves. Half the Al-Anon members—wives of alcoholics—in a West Coast city came from families with an alcoholic parent.[5] In addition, daughters of alcoholics become alcoholic 20–50 percent of the time. There seems to be a compelling need to repeat the patterns of their own families when they were growing up.

But as evidence that alcoholism may not be due to environment alone, one study showed that adopted women whose biological mothers were alcoholic were four times as likely to become alcoholic as those whose "real" mothers did not have a drinking problem.[6]

Is there any way to stem the compulsive rush toward repetition? At the Nassau County, New York, Alcohol Addiction Unit they think there is. Children of alcoholics, twelve years old and up, attend ten free sessions of group counseling. According to Dr. Joseph Kern, a psychologist and director of the unit, "Alcoholism is a family disease, but it doesn't have to be contagious. We try to get these children to see that they are important. Their lives can be salvaged. They can learn to live with themselves and with an alcoholic parent, too." It's too early to judge the success of the program, but by working with the husbands and wives of alcoholics as well as the children, they are optimistic they can step in and keep the alcoholic family from being a breeding ground for future problems.

As the Reverend Joseph L. Kellerman, the former director of the Charlotte, North Carolina, Council on Alcoholism, has been complaining for years, "We are so focused on playing savior to the sick that we forget our responsibility to the well."

Programs which recognize this responsibility will probably become more widespread. Now a New York State law allows alcohol-treatment facilities to deal with family members, even if the alcoholic herself is not in treatment.

Even when the alcoholic becomes sober, all the troubles may not disappear. Counselors have found that "the beginning of treatment is a shaky period, even after the drinking has stopped. If one of the partners in a marriage changes, and the other doesn't, it's hard to make it work." Sometimes there is an investment in keeping the alcoholic in the sick role; the others have forged a way to survive and resist any attempt to change what has become a familiar pattern. "It wasn't easy," a high school senior says, "for me to let my mother take charge of the kitchen again. I thought of it as my territory." Sometimes the marriage does not survive sobriety.

There are other disastrous social consequences of alcohol use and abuse. According to government figures, alcohol is associated with 50 percent of all murders (most murders involve family members or friends), more than 70 percent of all assaults, half of all rapes, 30 percent of all suicides, and half the fatal automobile accidents in the United States. One-third of the adult pedestrians who are fatally injured have blood-alcohol levels at or above legal intoxication. In England, a dozen deaths and 250 injuries each week have been attributed to drunken pedestrians. In this country, alcohol's misuse is estimated to cost society nearly $120 billion annually in lost production, health and medical costs, property damage, and welfare and criminal justice expenses. In New Jersey alone, more than half of all juvenile crime is said to be related to alcohol abuse. No one has put a dollar value on the damage to the family.

After this appalling litany, it's important to remember that 90 percent of the people who drink don't abuse alcohol and derive more pleasure than pain from its use. That prolific author Anonymous said it long ago with, "God, in his goodness, sent the grape." The problem for most families is not alcoholism, but how to encourage responsible drinking. "Drink the way you would like your children to drink. They learn from you," is the suggestion of Judith Seixas, a psychologist who developed a pioneering alcohol-abuse prevention program in suburban New York State. Dr. Chafetz believes alcohol shouldn't be mysterious or forbidden—parents should let children have a taste if they request it, and it should later be incorporated casually into meals. Studies have shown that the best predictor of a child's drinking habits is the drinking pattern of his or her parents—and mothers seem to have more influence than fathers. When a child reaches the teen years, however, friends are a lot more important than parents in setting the drinking pace.[7]

Most of the education for drinking in our society goes on without formal instruction, and if rising rates of teen-age drunkenness are any indication (in England, the number of girls found guilty increased 77 percent between 1964 and 1973), this method has not been particularly effective. At a symposium on drinking at Notre Dame University in South Bend, Indiana, student Diana Merten complained, "If you look at American society, two things are told to young adults; one is that you can't drink until you are eighteen or twenty-one, and the next thing you hear is that you can drink because you are eighteen or twenty-one. In between no one tells you how, or why, or where, or with whom. There is no institution in our society that has taken it upon itself to introduce young people to alcohol. Most families do not do it. Students are forced to drink behind closed doors or to sneak it out, or parents must lock up their liquor cabinets and things like that. All this does is form a real mystique about drinking."

For youngsters who tend to abuse substances, alcohol is still the "no-hassle drug." "The greatest cover is to get high on other drugs and drink a beer," a Dade County, Florida, teen-ager in a drug-abuse program reports. "Your mother smells alcohol, says 'okay, sleep it off.' She never guesses." That alcohol is the drug of choice for parents creates other problems for youngsters. They feel caught in a hypocritical contradiction; their parents tell them to stay away from drugs, yet are heavy users of alcohol and tranquilizers. When a survey on drug usage asked about use at home—including alcohol—this section was often left blank. "I can't handle that," was a common response. "I don't want to see that my parents use a drug." Parents are often unwilling to see how much youngsters are drinking—they might be forced to look at their own intake.

The conflicting messages—alcohol is a civilized addition to enjoyment; alcohol is a drug like any other—make it hard for families to deal with it clearly and consistently. Society's ancient ambivalence about alcohol once again complicates its use and abuse.

9

Alcohol and Pregnancy

*L*ife in the womb is traditionally idealized as the perfect state we're always trying to regain. There, cradled in warm fluid, we spend nine months protected by the placenta from the evils of the outside world, all our needs perfectly cared for. The trouble is that this vision doesn't stand up to the physiological facts of life. At least as far as alcohol is concerned, the placental barrier is a myth. Alcohol crosses the placenta to reach the fetus' bloodstream in about the same concentrations as in the mother's. When a mother drinks, the fetus drinks, too. When she drinks too much, she assaults her developing baby with a toxic drug whose effects cannot yet be fully calculated.

In 1973 Drs. Kenneth L. Jones and David W. Smith identified a cluster of birth defects they called the Fetal Alcohol Syndrome (FAS).[1] In the decade that followed, skepticism gave way to concern as evidence mounted that heavy drinking—five to six drinks a day—during pregnancy could result in clearly identifiable damage to the fetus. The damage appears most frequently in three areas: growth retardation, damage to the central nervous system (including mental retardation), and recognizable facial abnormalities such as small heads and flattened facial features. Heart and kidney abnormalities may also show up. For the woman who drinks heavily during pregnancy, the chances that she will have a malformed or retarded baby are reported to be greater than those for a woman who gets German measles early in pregnancy.

In 1984 Dr. Ann Streissguth and her colleagues at the University of Washington in Seattle reported that studies of the original FAS children followed through the years revealed that heart difficulties noticed at birth were not serious later, but that skeletal problems persisted. As for intelligence, although some had been diagnosed initially as severely retarded, their IQs often took such leaps that a few eventually came close to normal range, although none reached it. Commented Dr. Streissguth: "We believe the most long-term and devastating effects of alcohol are on the central nervous system." And even the best possible care after birth cannot erase the damage. Other studies have shown that 44 percent of the babies born to alcoholic women have average IQs of eighty, while an average IQ is one hundred.

FAS is, according to Dr. Ernest Noble, "the third leading known cause of mental retardation in this country, and the only one we know how to prevent." An estimated one to three of every thousand live births is an FAS child.

This startling number is a statistical guess, but doctors agree that alcohol causes harm much more often than anyone had thought. In recognition of this, Dr. Smith commented early in his research, "It just kills me when I see another affected child . . . and I know that if the mother had only known and stopped, it would not have happened. For most of the mothers of these babies it has been a crushing blow to find out that their drinking is why the baby has the problem."

FAS isn't the only problem of drinking and pregnancy. Several studies show that chances of a miscarriage go up in direct proportion to the amount of alcohol a mother drinks while she's pregnant. Even the moderate amount of two drinks a week is associated with a rise in the rate of spontaneous abortion (miscarriage). Drinking during late pregnancy presents dangers, too. It was once thought that alcohol during the third trimester would not affect the unborn baby, but the fetal brain goes through a growth spurt at that stage (and for months after birth), and even one session of drinking a few cocktails and some wine, without getting drunk, may be risky, according to a study presented at the

68th meeting of the Federation of American Societies for Experimental Biology. The researchers also warned that nursing mothers who drink could permanently harm the brain development of their children.

An accumulation of such studies prompted the Surgeon General of the United States to warn women "who are pregnant (or considering pregnancy) not to drink alcoholic beverages and to be aware of the alcoholic content of foods and drugs." Not drinking at all is the only way to be certain of safety.

How does alcohol cause problems? One possibility is that it directly affects the developing central nervous system of the fetus. Another is that acetaldehyde—the first breakdown product of alcohol metabolism and a potent poison—damages the developing cells. Clear damage to the fetus has been demonstrated in animal studies that can be controlled for diet, stress, genetics, and other factors that are difficult to measure in humans.

Dr. M. H. Kaufman, an anatomist at Cambridge University, England, has a hypothesis about the way alcohol may cause miscarriages. When he gave recently fertilized mice an amount of alcohol equivalent to what a woman might drink at a party, the eggs that would have become females showed a large percentage of chromosomal abnormalities. He warned that anything causing such abnormalities might give rise to spontaneous abortions (since the body is likely to reject faulty fetuses) even after only one drinking episode shortly after conception. Another possibility is that alcohol, by interfering with blood circulation through the umbilical cord, deprives the fetal brain of oxygen, causing brain damage that results in mental retardation. Dr. Anil B. Mukherjee and her colleagues at the National Institute of Child and Human Development found this kind of damage in infant monkeys even after their mothers had had only one "brief exposure" to alcohol.[2]

The question of exactly how much alcohol is necessary to do any harm is a matter of controversy. Dr. Henry Rosett and his colleagues at Boston City Hospital studied 469 pregnant women and their babies, but found effects only in the offspring of women who were sustained heavy drinkers. He believes that in studies showing damage at lower levels the women underreported their real drinking. On the other hand, researchers at the National Institute of Child Health and Human Development in Bethesda, Maryland, found in a study of thirty thousand mostly white, married, highly educated women that the more a mother drank the more likely she was to have an underweight baby, even though it was not premature. This was true for those who had less than one drink a day across the spectrum to those who had six or more drinks a day. Dr. James Mills, a pediatrician involved in the study, commented that "weight at birth is an extremely important marker for a baby's well-being. We are concerned that alcohol is causing some ill effect—as yet undetermined—on the fetus."[3]

Dr. Streissguth and her colleagues, too, found that even social drinkers could have babies who showed subtle changes (chiefly affecting the central nervous system) at birth, and even as late as the age of seven, these children had problems with attention span. Not all babies exposed to alcohol showed these effects, of course, but in a large sample she found a clear, worrisome relationship—"the more alcohol, the more damage." Before evidence of alcohol's influence on the fetal brain, these children who couldn't sit still, constantly interrupted, and just couldn't learn despite normal intelligence had been labeled everything from hyperkinetic to minimally brain damaged. There have been half a dozen attempts to account for the roughly 10 percent of American schoolchildren who exhibit these traits and none of them has been widely accepted. Whether alcohol will prove to be responsible remains to be seen.

As Dr. Streissguth sees it, however, there is a need for a category to encompass the less striking collection of subtle symptoms of alcohol-induced damage during pregnancy. She and others have proposed that these be called Fetal Alcohol Effects. One hopeful finding is that if a mother cuts down her drinking by mid-pregnancy, the harmful effects are diminished.[4]

If a mother continues drinking heavily right up to the time of birth, her baby may be born drunk and may suffer the tremors and convulsions of the D.T.'s—withdrawal symptoms as agonizing and threatening as the methadone- and heroin-withdrawal syndromes reported in the babies of drug addicts. There have been cases in which the amniotic fluid smelled of alcohol and the blood-alcohol level of the newborn baby was higher—and stayed high longer—than that of its drunken mother. There is speculation that this exposure to alcohol in the womb may predispose the infant to alcoholism in later life; the same kind of concern is now expressed about sensitizing infants to later allergic reactions by very early feeding of solid foods.

Dr. David Abramson studied infants with withdrawal tremors and liver damage at the Georgetown University Hospital. "In the forty weeks of gestation [one] can become an alcoholic, a true alcoholic with physical withdrawal," he says. "Is this baby a setup for alcoholism when he or she starts drinking socially at sixteen or seventeen?" Some of Dr. Abramson's babies, born to well-nourished middle-class mothers, had to be weaned gradually from their alcohol addiction, first intravenously and then by adding small quantities of alcohol to their milk.

Skeptics point out that many of the studies of birth anomalies and brain damage are based on samples of mostly impoverished women, and that women who drink heavily are also likely to smoke heavily and drink a lot of coffee. How can you be sure it's the alcohol and not malnutrition, nicotine, or caffeine that is causing the problems? Dr. Rosett concedes that it may take a combination of alcohol and malnutrition—his studies have been mostly on poor patients—but insists that alcohol is the chief culprit. A pilot project at the University of Florida College of Medicine has given preliminary support to this thesis.

Dr. Carrie Randall, a young neurochemist, became interested in the question of whether poor diet, nicotine, or high alcohol intake produced the malformed infants reported by other researchers. Of course, it was impossible to do a controlled experiment on human beings; but a strain of mice was available whose heredity and diet could be manipulated to remove any question about what led to any anomalies that might show up. Mice were impregnated and the experimental group was fed a completely adequate liquid diet with 25 percent of the calories as alcohol. The control group got the same diet, with 25 percent of the calories as sucrose (sugar). After nineteen days of gestation the fetuses were examined and photographed. The results were shocking. Fifteen of the sixteen litters of alcohol-fed mice had at least one malformed member. Only two of the control litters showed any abnormalities. Most frightening of all, the abnormalities—stunted limbs, enlarged heads, heart-valve damage—resembled those found in the victims of Thalidomide, a drug taken innocently by pregnant women in Europe in the 1960s. There is no question, Dr. Randall concluded, "that ethanol rather than malnutrition is the teratogenic agent."

In other words, at least in mice, it is alcohol, not poor diet, that produces the changes. It remains to be seen if more careful studies provide the same clear-cut evidence of cause and effect in human beings.

If alcohol does cause malformations, why haven't they shown up in large numbers? Maybe, the researchers in this field speculate, they just haven't been looked for. It took a long time to establish a relationship between lung cancer and smoking, but once the pattern was noticed, reports started piling up. There is also evidence that the effects may not show up at birth, but become obvious as growth slows to below normal during the first few years. Certainly not all babies of alcoholic mothers show all the disturbing anomalies. But they are generally lighter and shorter than other infants. A young woman who was alcoholic during her first pregnancies says, "I never thought about it at the time. But all of my babies were premature weight; full term, but all premature weight. With that last child, though, I couldn't drink much. I was very, very sickly. And—he was the biggest weight."

There is the first glimmer of evidence that even moderate doses of alcohol have damaging effects, particularly in the early months. Large-scale studies are now being conducted in Seattle, Boston, and Loma Linda, California, to verify this possibility. But there is no question that women who drink moderately have babies with lower than expected birth weights, like the babies of women who smoke. One struggling college student wailed when she learned of these studies, "Do you mean I could have been a genius if my mother hadn't had anything to drink when she was pregnant?"

No one will ever know what might have been for her, but Dr. LeClair Bissell, formerly the chief of New York's Roosevelt Hospital alcoholism treatment unit, says, "We don't know everything, but we know enough to tell a pregnant woman to cut out drinking entirely. We use the same precaution with any drug whose effects in pregnancy have not been rigorously tested. To be absolutely safe, she should stop drinking as soon as she decides to try to have a child."

Curiously, even without a doctor's advice, women seem to cut down on their alcohol consumption during pregnancy. In a study of 156 women by Ruth E. Little and Francia A. Shultz of the Johns Hopkins School of Medicine, average alcohol consumption dropped to less than half during pregnancy. Even monkeys and pigs on whom experiments have been conducted reduce their drinking during pregnancy.

These researchers uncovered the fact that women who are heavy drinkers concealed their drinking from their obstetricians, despite careful prenatal questioning. "Thus," Dr. Little says, "the person whose drinking may be doing the greatest harm is least likely to report it." In an attempt to get around this, Dr. Rosett of Boston City Hospital has experimented with the amino-acid test for heavy drinking (developed by Dr. Charles Lieber) on a sample of women coming to his prenatal clinic. He hopes to be able to identify chronic alcoholics without depending on their own notoriously inaccurate statements. Another doctor at Baltimore City Hospital in Baltimore recommends abortion during the first tri-mester if he is aware of a patient's heavy drinking. He has the same policy for a woman who has contracted German measles during that time.

The devastating recent reports on the results of heavy drinking during pregnancy were hailed as new observations. The embarrassing truth is they had been made and ignored, made again and discounted, through the ages. Of course, the early accounts don't stand up under modern scientific scrutiny, but that doesn't make them any less accurate as descriptions of what perceptive people had noticed. Mankind—and womankind—has been drinking alcohol and bearing children since prehistoric times. Aristotle warned, "Foolish, drunken, or hare-brained women, most part bring forth children like themselves," and Plato recommended that newly married couples who wanted to conceive should avoid intoxication.

Even the anomalies described by Smith and Jones were in the medical literature 200 years ago during England's disastrous gin epidemic. In 1720 the English government lifted restrictions on distilling and made it cheaper to buy gin than beer in order to help grain farmers make a profit. The epidemic of drunkenness that resulted hit hardest, not at the adults, but at those under five. It also lowered the birthrate. "Such [infants] as are born [are] meagre and sickly and unable to pass through the first stages of life"; they "often look shriveled and old," a committee of the Middlesex, England, Sessions reported in 1736.

A few years later, William Hogarth published his horrifying prints of Gin Lane. One of the most vivid, now in the Boston Museum of Fine Arts, shows a baby tumbling from its drunken mother's breast and another child being beaten. Later researchers have agreed with these early observers that it was excessive use of gin that caused fetal deaths and an upsurge in infant mortality; wages and crops were good and epidemic disease relatively rare.

Of course it can be argued that drunken parents neglect and mistreat their children, and that the mortality rate had little to do with the direct effect of alcohol on the fetus. And yet today's studies show that the infants of women who drink heavily have a newborn death rate of 17 percent compared with a 2 percent normal rate, and that almost half the children born to alcoholic mothers start life with some physical disability.[5]

When Rebecca H. Warner and Dr. Rosett of the Boston University School of Medicine surveyed the English and American literature on the effects of alcohol on offspring, they found that the ambivalence that haunts the entire field of alcohol research comes through most vividly when this touchy subject is approached. Warily, it has been asserted and then denied that alcohol does damage. Scientific attitudes are obviously not immune to cultural fashion.

By 1900 it was generally recognized (again) that alcohol readily passes through the placenta and affects the fetus, and also passes into mother's milk. But Prohibition came along and effectively ended almost all scientific inquiry into the effects of alcohol on the human body. Liquor was illegal, would soon pass from the scene, and anyway, there was something not quite dignified about studying it. The early studies could be ignored because they had been tainted by attitudes in modern scientific disfavor: that acquired characteristics (such as susceptibility to alcohol) could be inherited, and that alcohol had some direct effect on the germ plasm. Temperance advocates who saw alcohol behind every abnormality during the nineteenth century also made the whole subject rife for ridicule. Charles Dickens had his fun in 1836 in *Pickwick Papers* when the case of Betsy Martin was reported at a temperance society meeting: "Widow, one child and one eye, but knows her mother drank bottled stout, and shouldn't wonder if that caused it."

Even the fact that the placenta was no barrier slipped into oblivion except for the observations of one woman scientist who doggedly reported in 1923 that "the placenta acts as a protective filter for many substances but alcohol is not one of these." And she added, "I think it is not an exaggeration to state that alcohol is a poison, and that the fetus of a chronic alcoholic mother is itself a chronic alcoholic, absorbing alcohol from the mother's blood and subsequently from her milk"—conclusions that have just recently been reaffirmed.

As late as 1955 Mark Keller of the Rutgers School of Alcohol Studies made an attempt once and for all to finish off the controversy. "The old notions about children of drunken parents being born defective can be cast aside," he wrote, "together with the idea that alcohol can directly irritate and injure the sex glands."

Now, of course, there is convincing evidence of fetal-alcohol syndrome. And in 1976, twenty-one years after what was to have been the last salvo in the battle, the prestigious New England Journal of Medicine reported on studies showing that testosterone levels—even in normal men drinking alcohol for a short time—were reduced.[6] Alcoholism in men resulted in feminization, impotence, and sterility. In light of these and other corroborative findings, Dr. David Van Theil of the University of Pittsburgh School of Medicine asked his colleagues at a National Council on Alcoholism forum, "Does this mean that a man with low fertility shouldn't drink if he wants to father a child?" The New England Journal asked an equally haunting question: "Does alcohol diminish sexual function in woman?" No one yet knows, but someday we may find that ancient wisdom was right again—in the Old Testament Samson's mother is counseled by an angel, "Behold now, thou art barren, and bearest not; but thou shalt conceive and bear a son. Now therefore beware, I pray thee, and drink not wine nor any strong drink, and eat not any unclean thing." (Judges 13:7)

Dr. LeClair Bissell wondered for years why she saw so few pregnant alcoholic women; other doctors have been struck by the same phenomenon. When Sharon Wilsnack, a psychologist then at Harvard, looked into the childbearing histories of a limited sample of alcoholic and nonalcoholic women, she found that only 25 percent of the married alcoholics who had wanted children had succeeded. In one test group none of the heavy drinkers had been able to conceive. Later studies have confirmed that alcohol causes infertility, absent or reduced menstruation, and a loss of fat deposits in the breasts and hips— a "defeminization" comparable to the feminization that occurs in men. Both are due to alcohol's effects on the brain and pituitary gland, the regulators of hormone production. That alcohol doesn't interfere entirely with male and female fertility has been obvious through the ages; the stereotypically large families of drunken parents aren't just the invention of novelists.

Obviously, the study of alcohol's effects on the body is in its infancy, a bad pun but an accurate reflection on what is known so far. Since alcohol is water-soluble it reaches into almost every tissue, including the developing fetus and the organs that make it possible for conception to occur. Exactly what it does is still a matter for conjecture and controversy, but there is now compelling evidence that, as Dr. Noble put it, "The news is not good."

It is not all bad, either. Given our present understanding of alcohol's effect on the fetus, we finally know how to prevent a leading cause of mental retardation.

10

Treatment of Alcoholism

A lcoholism isn't simply an illness. It is a stigma kept hidden
by family and friends, even by hospitals and doctors. It is a
social disease that is misunderstood, ignored, and mis-
treated for the kindest of reasons. "My best friend is killing herself
with her drinking," one woman said, "but I can't say anything because I don't want to hurt her feelings." Alcohol is seldom implicated in the diagnosis of the 20–50 percent of all hospital patients
who are actually being treated for its consequences, particularly if
they are middle- and upper-class.

It is a condition that is whispered about, as breast cancer and
tuberculosis used to be, although it is this nation's third most common cause of death in people between thirty-five and fifty-five.
The conspiracy of silence keeps an estimated 95 percent of its victims undiagnosed and untreated until many have lost the stable
families that make successful treatment most likely. And yet, Dr.
Ernest Noble says, "Alcoholism is treatable, and a high recovery
rate is possible."

But as Dr. Frank Seixas, for nine years medical director of the
National Council on Alcoholism, relentlessly points out, "Treating
the alcoholic is like a recipe for rabbit stew: The first step is to
catch the rabbit." And that is not easy, particularly when women
are involved. Sociologists estimate that more than 70 percent of

the approximately 3.5 million alcoholic women in this country go untreated; only the skid-row derelict is readily identified. Other women are hidden or hide themselves. And Winnie Fraser of Canada's Addiction Research Foundation says, "From discussions with many women, I think it's the stigma that is keeping them hidden." (Drug and alcoholism counseling centers in Missouri are located in real-estate offices and next to fast-food franchises to assure women that no one will guess they are coming for treatment.)

Coupled with society's pervasive attitude that a woman who is alcoholic has fallen off her pedestal and failed as a woman, wife, and mother, there is the woman's own denial that she could be "like the bum in the street"—the stereotyped legacy of the temperance movement that is still powerfully with us.

A Midwestern teacher says, "I kept telling myself I couldn't be alcoholic. Here I was, teaching and getting my master's degree and smarter than most other people. If I could do all that, I couldn't be alcoholic." Others tell themselves they don't fit the label because they drink only wine, or keep their houses spotless, or don't miss more work than anyone else. This puzzling persistence in the face of reality—"Why can't they admit how sick they're getting?"—is seen by one experienced counselor as a part of the illness: "The sicker they get, the less capable they are of recognizing the nature of the illness or its severity."

Self-protective denial, an unconscious mechanism, sometimes reaches incredible proportions. A New York doctor who specializes in the treatment of alcoholism has seen "an intelligent patient, with a drink in hand, tell me he had not had a drink for two weeks. This would be lying if the patient didn't believe it himself."

Some women are helped to perpetuate the denial by husbands who can't bear to think of their wives as anything by social drinkers or who minimize the problem because "somebody has to take care of the house and kids." "I was rescued until I was almost dead," a cherub-faced, recovered alcoholic recalled. "When my husband walked out on me finally, that was good for me. Unless an alcoholic can experience the consequences of drinking . . . as long as we're protected from our own crises, we won't make it."

Then there are the employers who are embarrassed to confront their female workers about their absences. "Female complaints" are still a good cover-up. For the drinker herself, the denial may not be just a psychological defense. Alcoholic blackouts effectively erase the memory of how much was consumed and what happened afterwards; even when the drinker does recall the events of the night before she is likely to see them through euphoric eyes: "What do you mean I talked nonstop? I really made some good points and put him in his place." She is not lying; she really remembers it this way.

The only thing that cuts through this web of "I'm not having any real problems" or "I can quit anytime I want to" is some sort of crisis. For women, the crisis is often centered in the family.

After years of patiently making excuses when his wife passed out before dinner guests arrived, one big-city lawyer finally told her, "I'm taking you to the best treatment facility around, and then I'm leaving. I've found out that I have a right to some happiness, too."

A young mother walked into an outpatient treatment unit the day after she'd spent an hour searching for her two-year-old son. She'd left him in the wrong car in a parking lot while she went back to the supermarket for a minute.

Physical difficulties are another crisis area. Even when there isn't a medical emergency, women will finally admit to their alcoholism when they become "sick and tired of feeling sick and tired." One businesswoman told her counselor that she would throw up every day, then drag herself to work. But she kept getting whatever illness was around, such as flu and bronchitis (excessive alcohol intake lowers immunity), and finally couldn't shake the illnesses. Even the tea laced with brandy that she drank to ease her discomfort didn't work any more.

Then there are the psychological crises. "I was in an absolute panic. I was afraid I was losing my mind," is how one housewife put it. "My father had killed himself, and I was having all kinds of morbid thoughts."

The theory used to be that an alcoholic had to hit bottom before she could accept help, and bottom often meant a wrecked marriage, no job, the end of the road. The attitude was, "The alcoholic has to admit it and ask for help; nobody can do it for her." This has now been successfully disputed by people such as Dr. Vernon Johnson of the Johnson Institute in Minneapolis. He says, "It is unconscionable and unnecessary for an alcoholic to hit bottom. Interventions do work, and we can intervene much earlier than was thought if we have the data from people who have first-hand knowledge."

What Dr. Johnson and the hundreds of people his institute has trained suggest is this: Make use of the crises that are part of every alcoholic's life. Bring together two or three people to read aloud specific lists of how the alcoholic has behaved. Confront her without anger, but with concern. And the denial will drop away.

"Last night you fell asleep in the chair and burned a hole in the arm. It was lucky I walked in and kept the whole thing from going up in flames."

"You couldn't stand up and get out of the car after the Carlsons' party."

"When my friends were here Saturday night you promised to bake a cake. You never did."

This kind of buildup of reality, says Dr. Johnson, helps an alcoholic come to the realization that she is hurting more people than she ever imagined and needs help. The relentless listing of events—not hearsay—harnesses the alcoholic's guilt and makes it harder to hide from responsibility. Dr. Johnson, an Episcopal minister, uses the story of the Garden of Eden to illustrate this mechanism. God finds Adam, even though he tries to hide. And the evasion of blame, "which apparently began with Adam," commences: "She made me do it." And for Eve: "It was the serpent." They both, finally, have to face the real consequences of their action.

The connection of the story of the fall of man with the use of alcohol goes back into the dim recesses of history. There is a Talmudic commentary (B. Sanhedrin, 478) that suggests the forbidden fruit was not an apple, but a bunch of grapes, "for only wine brings woe." Confronting the drinker with this woe sometimes breaks down the walls of resistance.

Often, even without the skilled rehearsals and support that Dr. Johnson's institute offers to family and friends, concerned observers can push an alcoholic into reality. Jan Clayton, the actress, remembered that "a light went on in my head when I found a letter in my mailbox from Alcoholics Anonymous, saying my friends were concerned about me."

Of course, the denial doesn't stop with the first reach for help; it may take a long time for a problem drinker to accept the central role of alcohol in her life. As Dr. LeClair Bissell, head of the Smithers Center in New York for years, said wryly, "We didn't have any alcoholics coming in. They just become alcoholics after we'd been treating them for a while."

It's not only the alcoholic who has trouble seeing herself clearly. Law enforcement officials tend to look the other way when a woman, not a man, is involved in a drunk-driving incident. Unless there is verbal abuse or someone else has been hurt, the police are likely just to drive the woman home. "While apparently favorable to women in the short run," comments Dr. Milton Argeriou, who conducted a study of drunk-driving arrests in Boston, "it may well be deleterious if it results in aiding problem-drinking women to keep their problems hidden."

If policemen and judges are reluctant to identify a woman as alcoholic—the pedestal again—doctors, counselors, and other professionals are equally protective—or blind. Dr. Ephraim T. Lisansky of the University of Maryland chided his colleagues for missing the diagnosis of alcoholism, reminding them that "most of us who are health professionals come from a certain segment of the population which does not accept alcoholism as a disease, but as a misbehavior." Since as doctors and nurses they aren't looking for sin but for symptoms, they pass by the evidence.

Dr. Lawrence I. Senseman tried to help his fellow physicians overcome their myopia when he wrote "The Housewife's Secret Illness: How to Recognize the Female Alcoholic." From his years of experience in a sanatorium for middle-class alcoholics he warned, "She can be a most convincing fabricator, but fortunately she is only deceiving herself, using the mechanism of denial." He suggests that doctors be suspicious of the woman who reaches for a cigarette with shaky hands or who has scars on her arms, the result of burns from the walls of the oven. Picking up on the "Magnolia Blossom syndrome" noticed by many other investigators, he reports, "Her manner may be suspiciously demure, with a soft voice, fluttery eyes, and a tendency toward being overcooperative." She may also smell of alcohol underneath the disguise of mouthwash, breath fresheners, or perfume.

Even when he is faced with these warning signs, the doctor is often unwilling to press his patient for a drinking history. "It is all too easy for the physician to regard as utterly preposterous," Dr. Senseman continues, "the notion that the gray-haired pleasant lady in his office, perhaps the staid town librarian or the minister's wife, is an alcoholic."

It is equally hard for the woman to see herself that way, and many alcoholics are consummate con artists. They talk about headaches, or lack of sleep, or nervousness, never mentioning their drinking. In Kentucky, members of the local National Council on Alcoholism Task Force on Women and Alcohol put these posters in doctor's offices: "Is your nerves problem really a drinking problem?" Often the doctor, as a person dedicated to relieving pain, prescribes a tranquilizer for the "nerves," and the woman is soon doubly addicted—to Valium or Librium plus alcohol. The National Institute on Drug Abuse estimates that twice as many women as men use tranquilizers. A Maryland women's task force is trying to convince doctors that "alcoholism in women is not a Librium deficiency." But it is a hard fight. Since women are more likely to turn up in doctor's offices, and doctors more often prescribe mood-changing drugs for them, this double burden is theirs more often than it is men's. Many women also use amphetamines ("speed") for weight reduction or to treat hangovers, and are caught in another addiction.

The doctor who persists in trying to understand what is behind his patient's complaints may also be in trouble. Herbert Cooper, a Massachusetts gastroenterologist whose patients' conditions are often caused or aggravated by alcohol, laments, "I haven't yet found any way to ask a woman about her drinking and get an honest answer. With a man it's different. He may look a little shamefaced and say, 'Well, you know how it is. I shouldn't smoke so much, either.' If things are bad enough, the woman's husband or one of the children may talk to me privately and tell me she has a problem with liquor."

In an attempt to get honest answers from alcoholics who fool themselves as well as doctors, psychiatrists at Glasgow University, Scotland, tried two approaches: In one, psychiatrists asked the questions; in the other, a computer asked the same questions (they were displayed on a screen, and the patients—all men—pushed buttons to indicate their answers). When they worked the computer, the men admitted to 30 percent more drinking than when they were face-to-face with another human being. Notoriously lacking in trust, the alcoholics evidently felt more comfortable and freer to reveal themselves to a machine. The Scottish experts sug-

gest it might be worthwhile to have computers available at selected health centers to speed up early identification.

Women with drinking problems are less obvious than men.
Some of them are in the traditional women's jobs—as teachers, social workers, nurses, beauticians—and, without special attempts
to reach them, are largely ignored. But in at least one industrial
treatment program, women outnumber men three to one, even
though there are more male employees. Why? Because there was a
direct outreach to women, with a note enclosed in pay envelopes
that said of alcoholism, "Women are not immune." A labor expert
with New York State's Division of Alcoholism says, "Many women
thought the employer had sent the letter just to them."

Is there any way to find the alcoholic who doesn't work, doesn't
talk to a doctor about her drinking, and who hides at home? Television has been tried. "I've gotten requests for help after a morning show when I said, 'All right. You've got the ironing board out
and the bottle. Let's talk,' " actress Jan Clayton reported. There
have been other original ideas. One counselor suggests this untra-
ditional way to get a message inside the front door: train Tupper-
ware hostesses, Avon Ladies, and Welcome Wagon greeters in the
techniques of talking to a woman who drinks too much, then send
them into homes with "soap, perfume, deodorants, and lots of
literature." The approach would reach some "unaffiliated"
women—those who don't even belong to the PTA. That parents'
organization, too, would be a good place to reach women. A study
of AA members by Jane E. James showed that 60 percent of them
were PTA members during their drinking years.

The traditional women's clubs are being enlisted, too, in the
search for those who need treatment. "These organizations have
been active and effective in many other problem areas. Now
we're involving them in the area of alcohol abuse," says Jan Du-
Plain, who started the office on women of the National Council
on Alcoholism. And the importance of this problem in women's
lives was brought vividly to life at the 1977 Houston Conference
on Women when shirts and buttons reading "Alcoholism is a
Woman's Issue" appeared at the meetings. As one feminist emphasized, "We've come to the conclusion that alcoholism is an
equal-opportunity disease, and we're asking for equal opportunity
to recover."

Women are usually underrepresented in public treatment programs; in California, there are four men to every woman. Some private programs, however, report as many women as men in treatment.

Treatment for alcoholism, once it has been identified, takes place in a variety of settings: a doctor's office, a clinic, a general or psychiatric hospital, a facility set up specifically to handle alcoholics—but the ways the problem is approached fall into a few specific areas:

Physical

The alcoholic woman who is brought to a hospital or "drying out" facility by family (rarely her husband) or friends is desperately in need of medical attention. First, of course, she must be withdrawn from alcohol (and often drugs) and protected from the sometimes fatal effects of delirium tremens—the D.T.'s. Less serious withdrawal symptoms of anxiety and shakiness can be controlled by minor tranquilizers—Librium, Valium, or some similar drug, commonly used to diminish tension. For most patients, these are discontinued a few days before discharge so that the patient can go on to other treatment free from the haze of chemicals. Some doctors (in private practice or treatment facilities) continue to prescribe so-called "minor" tranquilizers to ease their alcoholic patients back into normal living. But one experienced physician emphasizes, "This may be a question of today's treatment becoming tomorrow's problem." Dr. LeClair Bissell, a recovered alcoholic herself, is strongly against the long-term use of these drugs. "Alcoholics," she points out, "are people prone to seek a chemical solution to human problems. Why then would anyone want to risk compounding their difficulties by giving them yet another addicting drug?" What doctors call "major" tranquilizers are another matter. These nonaddictive drugs, prescribed for schizophrenics (who may also be alcoholic), may be lifesaving when used on a long-term basis to treat psychoses.

In a hospital setting or on an outpatient basis, patients are given vitamin B_1 (to reverse some of the ravages of alcohol in the body) and other vitamins to supplement an often inadequate diet, and are treated for whatever other physical problems they may have. Then they may be offered a drug to help them stay away from drinking.

These drugs—Antabuse (disulfiram, used in the United States) or Temposil (citrated calcium carbamide, used in Canada)—swiftly produce unpleasant effects if combined with drinking. Nausea, vomiting, a pounding headache, flushing, and an irregular heartbeat follow inexorably if a patient swallows or even inhales alcohol. The hope is that this kind of reaction, or even the fear of it, will keep a drinker from reaching for that first sip. It also insures a few days free of liquor to get other help. But Antabuse is tricky; when it was introduced thirty years ago a few patients died as a result of its interaction with alcohol. Now lower doses are generally prescribed and fewer untoward effects have been reported. Even with low doses, however, a person on Antabuse may have a severe reaction to "hidden" alcohol—in mouthwash, for instance, or in flavorings. That's why doctors agree these drugs should never be given without the patient's cooperation and informed consent. Doctors don't prescribe it for people with weak hearts or those who, for other reasons, might not withstand the reaction.

There is another problem with the drug. It is usually given daily (its effects last up to four days) by mouth. Sometimes a determined alcoholic will accept the dosage, then spit it out, hide it in her cheek, or take it home and not swallow it. To get around this, some treatment centers have patients swallow the dose (which has been dissolved in water) while someone watches. Even this doesn't always work; people have thrown up the dosage before it could be absorbed into the body. There are stories, too, of alcoholics who have worked out a secret way to take the drug yet escape the unpleasant consequences when they drink.

Like any other treatment method, Antabuse should be prescribed on an individual basis. This kind of deterrent seems to be more effective in older, more stable men and women who have been drinking for a long time but are not depressed. Young people are more likely to become depressed, stop taking it, and drop out of therapy.

In Denmark, where Dr. Erik Jacobsen first stumbled on Antabuse's interaction with alcohol, it is given to patients for 200 days, "so they can learn to live a nonalcoholic life. Antabuse is no cure. The real cure is the patient's reintegration of himself."

Dr. Ruth Fox, the New York psychiatrist who first introduced the drug into this country, used it for her patients for a quarter of a century with almost no significant side effects, even after years of regular use. The unpleasant consequences hit, of course, when the patient mixes Antabuse and alcohol. The anti-alcohol effects are interfered with, however, if a patient takes iron pills or Maalox, a common remedy for stomach discomfort.

For doctors in private practice, Antabuse is a difficult drug. Unless the patient comes in every day, there's no guarantee that she is actually swallowing her prescribed dosage. To get around this, there has been some experimentation with implanting Antabuse under the skin, so it is released slowly and requires only an occasional visit to the doctor. This method has not yet proven effective. As a matter of fact, when he reviewed the results of scientific studies on Antabuse and its effect on drinking, Dr. T. M. Kitson of New Zealand concluded: "Any success achieved by disulfiram therapy [Antabuse] (particularly involving implantation) is probably due more to psychological factors than to the [drug] itself." An American researcher put it more bluntly: "Antabuse is probably an active placebo; but for all practical purposes this is all we've got." In other words, it is hard to measure the effectiveness of the drug because it is hard to know if it has really been taken. Maybe what keeps people from drinking again is the *conviction* that it will make them sick; it doesn't actually have to be tested. Although it is the only thing (along with Temposil) specifically designed to treat alcoholism, a sugar pill might work as well. In the early days, doctors would put a patient on a test dosage of the drug under careful supervision, in their offices or in a hospital. Then, the patient would be given a slug of alcohol. The swift, acutely unpleasant results were counted on to keep the alcoholic from testing the drug on his own. Now, it is agreed, just detailing the reactions is enough.

Does it help? Dr. Fox and many others are convinced that it provides an extra reason for staying away from liquor when the alcoholic is just beginning to try to break her old patterns. At Rockland Psychiatric Center in New York State (and many other facilities), all patients in the alcoholic rehabilitation unit take the drug every day, unless there are medical reasons to avoid it. Other treatment facilities feel it is a crutch and, although they may accept its use at first, they try to wean the patient from it.

For a while it was hoped that another drug—one that produced pleasant rather than unpleasant effects—could help the alcoholic.

This was LSD (lysergic acid diethylamide), the psychedelic drug which produces visions and intense spiritual experiences in some people. It was used experimentally with what seemed like success; subjects reported greater insight into their problems and said they felt better able to stay away from alcohol. Later research, however, has not supported these early claims, and its use has been largely abandoned.

People Therapy

It's a truism that alcohol is a people substitute, and people are an alcohol substitute. The pervasive emotional tone of alcoholics is a despairing loneliness. Most formal programs and many private physicians and counselors recognize this and include the fellowship of Alcoholics Anonymous as part of the treatment process. AA began in Akron, Ohio, in 1935 when two sober alcoholics discovered they had better luck staying away from liquor when they helped other people with the same struggle. Now there are more than 476,000 men and women in the United States and Canada who agree that they are powerless over alcohol and that their fate is in the hands of a higher power. To some, that power is a traditional, religious God; to others, it is the group itself or some spiritual force to which they can turn. By bringing their common problem out into the open (meetings begin with: "My name is Jean [or Bill or Mary] and I'm an alcoholic"), they develop what an AA pamphlet calls a "sharing of experience, strength, and hope that seems to be the key element that makes it possible for them to live without alcohol and, in most cases, without even wanting to drink." As one member put it, "When you get rid of the booze, you need something to take its place, and what you have is AA."

AA is generally recognized as the most successful of the treatment approaches now available. Dr. Fox, a former medical director of the National Council on Alcoholism, says, "AA has undoubtedly reached more cases than all the rest of us [doctors] together. For patients who can and will accept AA it may be the only form of therapy needed." In large metropolitan areas there are meetings every night and during lunch hours, some of them specialized. There are women's groups, gay groups, professional groups, blue-collar groups. Experienced AA watchers can characterize them by socioeconomic status, the depth of the religious feeling, ethnicity. Many meet in churches and end their meetings with the Lord's Prayer. Others meet in libraries or business buildings. There is a group to fill almost any need, and when more than one group is available, members are advised to shop around until they are comfortable.

Regular attendance helps a person understand and live by some of the AA bywords: "One day at a time" (no one can contemplate *never* drinking again) and "Take it easy" (often seen on bumper stickers). There is also the helping network of AA members, available by phone or in person to listen and offer support. Some chapters even have a Mayday squad whose members go out any time of the day or night to take someone to a hospital or treatment center or just to make a house call and help fight the urge to take that first drink.

But AA isn't for everyone. There are some people whose natural reticence makes it impossible for them to reveal themselves in a group. Some whose families are intact see themselves as different from others who have hit "bottom" and are essentially homeless and friendless. Wealthier alcoholics may feel that costly individual therapy protects their privacy and provides better treatment than they could get in a roomful of people talking about their problems with drinking. Of course, AA is often used in conjunction with other therapies. There is also a feeling that AA is largely middle class. One counselor at a halfway house for women who had spent time in prison said, "It isn't for street people."

The anonymity required by AA (only first names are used; members are asked not to identify themselves in print or on TV) has also been questioned. Since AA is dedicated to removing the stigma from alcoholism and to bringing the problem out into the open, Mercedes McCambridge says, "I argue with Alcoholics Anonymous about the word *anonymous*. I don't understand why that's necessary. Why is it 400,000 people in this country have to live with no name when their only crime is that they have a legal disease? They will tell you it is to protect the newcomer to their organization. Well, what are we protecting the newcomer from, from being known as an alcoholic? As a person with a legitimate disease? . . . Would you do that to a diabetic or an asthmatic?"

AA reaches only a small proportion of the people who suffer from Ms. McCambridge's "legal disease." This is partly because of the myths that hinder acceptance of its help. New York psychiatrist Stuart Nichols suggested that his colleagues were at fault in not referring their private patients to AA, feeling, as one of them said, "It's too religious and too authoritarian." If they would attend a few meetings, Dr. Nichols continued, they would find that in many cases the spiritual base is hardly evident and that even sophisticated patients can benefit from the understanding and support of other alcoholics. He conceded, however, that for some patients AA may not be the best thing.

One thing that isn't a myth is the reputation AA has for being a great place to meet single men. (At this point, one-third of all members are women—which means that two-thirds are men.) But this sometimes complicates progress. "I went right into another bad marriage with someone I met at meetings," a woman married four times recalls. "We were leaning on each other so hard neither of us had separate lives. We started drinking together, too."

To avoid some of the sexual tensions and provide a place for women to discuss their special problems out of earshot of men, there are now over 600 AA women's groups in the United States and Canada. In one of them a Midwestern thirty-year-old who had been in inpatient treatment for three weeks was finally able to talk about the terror she had hidden all this time because she was embarrassed to talk about it in front of men. During her withdrawal from alcohol she had begun to bleed vaginally. The bleeding had continued, and she was now afraid she was hemorrhaging, convinced there was something seriously wrong. She learned she was just suffering one of the aftereffects of withdrawal, and the bleeding quickly stopped with the correct medication.

Success rates are hard to evaluate. Scientists at New York's Downstate Medical Center question the validity of the figures released by AA itself because it has consistently refused to let itself be studied by an impartial outside source.[1] The anonymity of participants is zealously guarded. One study by John Norris, head of the AA Board of Directors, indicated that 25 percent of AA members have not had a drink for five years or more, and of these, 91 percent stayed sober in following years, particularly if they attended AA meetings regularly. These may seem like dismally low achievements, but when you consider that many doctors have found the usual approaches of exhortation, medication, and exploration don't work at all, they begin to seem remarkable.

Talking Therapies

All sorts of people try to help the alcoholic when she comes for treatment. They include doctors, ministers, social workers, psychologists, and alcoholism counselors—many of whom are recovered alcoholics. There is a feeling among helpers who deal with the social and psychological consequences rather than the medical ones that recovered alcoholics do the best job. But even this hallowed attitude is now being questioned. Bishop Walter Brown, who runs two long-term treatment facilities with both former alcoholics and nonalcoholics on his staff, says, "The recovering alcoholic is not always the best counselor. There's nobody so self-righteous as the recovering alcoholic—'My life was the same as yours, so you do like I did and you'll be fine.' They know all the answers. In this field, you have to know your limitations. All professions have a place."

Whatever their training, they all try to help the alcoholic understand herself and her drinking. For women in particular, there is a need in these one-to one sessions to mourn for the years they have lost and to weep about what might have been. In treating women alcoholics in a California outpatient clinic, social worker Penny Clemmons found that many therapists are unwilling to let this happen. "They tend to brush it off—they can't stand crying."

Once the mourning has been worked through, a woman is ready to enter the second phase of treatment, Ms. Clemmons says, and work on her guilt. "Particularly if there are children, there is a never-ending struggle to forgive oneself." It is in this second phase (which may begin in a few months, or not until a woman has been in treatment a year or more) that psychotherapy can take place, she believes.

Many counselors, once they have made clear the role alcohol plays in a patient's problems, turn the responsibility for recovery over to the person seeking help. "It is essential in treatment to understand you are never, ever going to sober anyone up. You can offer encouragement, the tool, but you are never going to do it for them. This attitude places the responsibility—and the credit—squarely with the patient," says one counselor and recovered alcoholic who helps women look at their drinking patterns and face the precipitating emotions that have propelled them into alcoholism. Most of them find they drink out of loneliness and self-hatred. "When they feel better about themselves," she adds, "they are less likely to reach for the bottle."

Doctors in private practice who treat alcoholics are often discouraged by the difficulties involved. "I've tried to treat them," one said. "It's not a disease. Keep them away from my door." In a national survey of physicians by sociologists Robert W. Jones and Alice R. Helrich, seven out of ten agreed that alcoholics are uncooperative and difficult patients. Yet psychiatrists like Ruth Fox have treated thousands successfully. She used a long initial interview in which she took a thorough drinking history and tried to educate her patients about alcohol's effects. They are usually abysmally misinformed. She then encouraged them to join one of her groups and also AA. "I was trained as a psychoanalyst," she says, "but I don't use it at all. Psychoanalysis is contraindicated in the treatment of alcoholism." The uncovering of deep, early problems, and the regression that is encouraged may be too stressful.

Several studies indicate that women do better in individual therapy than in groups.[2] This is dismissed as a "myth" by Ruth Sanchez Dirks, a social worker who was special assistant to the director at the National Institute on Alcohol Abuse and Alcoholism (NIAAA). "Treatment personnel carry their biases with them, but when they are accepting of women, group treatment works. The myth that a woman responds better in individual therapy may reflect her difficulties in mixed groups where she can't feel free to discuss sexual matters."

Individual treatment, of course, tries to help the patient stop drinking. Before he began seeing patients and advising them that abstinence was the only way to straighten out their lives, one New York doctor set aside one month during which he didn't drink at all. "It was a very difficult social experience," he reports. "We ought to understand what we're asking of our patients in this drinking society."

In some cases, getting the person to stop drinking is a "baby step." Therapists of all disciplines agree that the hard thing is getting the patient to develop relief systems. What can you offer to take the place of the rosy glow, the relief from anxiety, the hours spent in drinking with other people? "If you stand on your head for two hours in Times Square, it's okay if it makes you feel better," is what one psychiatrist tells his patients. Most don't go quite that far, but find renewed satisfactions, once sober, in family life or hobbies or further education. A Pennsylvania counselor said half-jokingly, "Our women provide half the freshman class for our local community college."

Women, more often than men, have asked for help in one way or another before they finally enter treatment aimed at their alcoholism. This is partly because women are more likely to use medical services than men. But they can also hide their drinking problem behind a host of other complaints. "I saw three psychiatrists before I got here," said one halfway house resident. "I conned them all. I'm the best faker of a neurosis you ever saw. I told one of them about my drinking, but lied about the amount. He thought I'd been sober for two weeks when it was really for two days." Most women have been drinking heavily for eleven years before they are treated for alcoholism itself.

In many cases, individual counseling is not enough, and most programs also include group therapy of one kind or another.

Group Therapies

Some group methods emphasize support and understanding. Others use the confrontational techniques developed in the treatment of drug addicts to break down defenses and leave patients more open to change. One professional woman who had been drinking for years and came from "a nicely decadent Southern family" found herself verbally assaulted by four-letter words when she told her group she saw herself as "a lady." "I soon learned that an alcoholic is an alcoholic and I'm no different from anyone else. That's when I could come to grips with my life."

Transactional analysis is a method that has adapted Freud's classic id, ego, and superego to a system which has each person include within herself a child, an adult, and a parent. These are constantly battling for control. Although all people play games and have a "script" they follow, sick people (alcoholics among them) play games in which they are more often the victims ("If it wasn't for my lousy marriage, I wouldn't be here"). Sometimes unraveling these patterns can be helpful in breaking the cycle of destructive drinking.

Psychodrama is another technique that is sometimes beneficial. In this, patients and therapist play family roles and uncover hidden conflicts that may be contributing to a drinking problem. At England's Accept day-care center for alcoholics, this technique prompted one member to say, "They really turn you inside out without you knowing."

More focused on the present, family therapy has come to be an important part of many treatment programs, particularly if family members (husbands, children, parents) are still in the picture. Unfortunately, by the time many alcoholics are involved in treatment, their families have effectively deserted them.

When families (or couples) do get together, they may be helped to see how the whole family system contributes to the alcoholic's problems. Sometimes alcohol plays a part in keeping them together, and this dimly perceived role makes it even more difficult to interfere with the drinking pattern. George Washington University researcher Peter Steinglass told of one couple who wasn't able to be physically close unless both partners were drunk. Family members may also cover up consequences, intensify the alcoholic's emotional isolation, or, for some reason, need to have a "sick" person to concentrate on. Talks of husband and wife or whole families with a therapist offer a way to restore a balance that has been disturbed by one person being "overfunctioning"— taking on more than his or her share—and the other being "underfunctioning." A surprising finding that has emerged from this approach is that the alcoholic can get better even if he or she never enters treatment. Both Dr. Murray Bowen, a pioneer in family systems theory, and Dr. LeClair Bissell report complete "cures" of serious drinking problems when only other family members attended the sessions. The alcoholic was never seen, but changing the family climate was enough to end the drinking. The best results, though, came when husband and wife were involved together.

One kind of group therapy that does require the alcoholic's presence is consciousness raising. Growing out of the women's movement, this is a technique often used to battle low self-esteem. At a state hospital inpatient program, one counselor has each participant take turns telling all the good things she can think of about herself. "I'm alive. . . . I'm kind." They soon get stuck, and any other group member is free to add, "You're beautiful," or to fantasize about her sister alcoholic—"I see you as a model in a black silky dress." One young woman said to an older one, "I see you as a suburban matron," and was greeted with laughter and the response, "I was born in Harlem." All the good things are written down, and each woman takes her own list back to post on her mirror. "These are realistic positives," the counselor explains, "and seeing them again and again helps a woman recognize that she has a lot of good going for her—and people who care about her."

Alcoholic women also have to be helped to deal with their anger. "Why me?" they want to know. And they are enraged (although they may not realize it) that they cannot have the pleasure of drinking again. They have often had trouble expressing anger in their lives; assertiveness training, learning to "speak up without being knocked down," helps them deal with feelings they may have subdued with alcohol when they were drinking.

There is an impression among some treatment personnel that women do better in all-women groups, with a woman leader. In one program, the percentage of women completing treatment rose from 35 percent to 59 percent when groups of this kind were started. When a man took over the women's group, only 38 percent of the patients stuck it out through the whole process. Other experts caution that a good therapist is a good therapist, regardless of sex. Dr. Sheila Blume said, "I've spent five years working with men-only groups, five with women only, and five with mixed—and they all worked. I think men can treat women, and women can treat men."

Reality Therapy

Although many other therapies are aimed at changing the internals—how a woman feels about herself—reality therapy is aimed at changing the conditions of her life. She is taught the facts about her alcoholism and the effect of alcohol on her body. Like diabetics, alcoholics who understand their disease are better able to cooperate in treatment. Surprisingly, they know less than other people about the drug they abuse. When they questioned heavy drinkers on New York's skid row, Drs. G. R. Garrett and H. M. Bahr found their answers "revealed an array of interesting, though mostly fictitious beliefs, about alcoholic beverages. One woman who claimed to have lived in the subways for sixteen years explained that she had avoided becoming an alcoholic by periodically switching brands and types of beverages."

Women in treatment are also given help in finding jobs, learning to take care of a home, and completing or beginning advanced schooling. "Reality is reality," a longtime counselor says flatly. "We can't worry too much about the women's movement and whether they're in stereotyped roles. These women are going to have to go out and take care of themselves and their families. They're going to have to cook and sew and do all the things women do who have husbands, and a lot of them without men in their lives are going to have to support themselves and their kids. Our job is to prepare them."

As a matter of fact, when Do It Now Foundation, devoted to working in the field of drug and alcohol abuse, surveyed treatment agencies, it found the women's movement had had no real effect on addicted women.[3] Probably the effect has been on those who do the treatment. It has certainly increased their awareness of women and their particular needs, and provided an impetus to examine staff ratios (are there enough women to treat the women who come?) and programs with inadequate provisions for women.

Behavior Therapy

This relatively new technique is used to produce either of two different results, abstinence or controlled drinking. The first—traditional abstinence—is encouraged by repeatedly giving alcoholics something that makes them throw up after every drink (in a hospital setting) or by making drinking unattractive by giving them an electrical shock every time they pick up a glass with alcohol in it. The theory is that such immediate results will teach the alcoholic that drinking is unpleasant and should be avoided. In one study alcoholics were given the drug apomorphine to produce nausea. Four years after treatment, 64 percent of the patients were still abstinent. But these "aversive conditioning" methods raise certain questions, even among those friendly to the theory behind them. Dr. E. J. Larkin of Canada's Addiction Research Foundation finds the results disappointing because "aversive conditioning replaces compulsive behavior with a phobia—clearly not the best of all possible events." The phobia, however, does not threaten life. The compulsive drinking does.

Flying in the face of conventional wisdom, behavior therapy has also been used to teach alcoholics to drink moderately, at least in the hospital. Some researchers have reinforced controlled drinking by rewarding it emotionally. The patient is praised, given certain privileges, and supported by other members of the group. Electric shock has been used by others to hold drinking down to acceptable limits instead of discouraging it completely.

Despite enthusiastic reports of success with these techniques (on men only), there has been criticism of studies which indicated improvement in the hospital but didn't provide careful follow-ups or control groups—comments that could be made about most alcoholism research. When Dr. Alfonso Paredes was at the University of Oklahoma Health Sciences Center, he had good luck teaching alcoholics to control their drinking, even when they were free to walk out of their hospital ward to a neighborhood bar. "But," he says gloomily, "many weren't able to maintain their control when they got out of the hospital and went right back into their old living situations. It may be," he speculates, "that many alcoholics knowingly or unknowingly use alcohol to avoid coping with assigned expectations, expectations that are temporarily suspended when they are admitted to a hospital and assume the patient role within the institutional setting. . . . The critical variables that induce deviant drinking, making it compulsive, redundant, and provocative, are just not there."

Proponents of the psychological school, which sees alcoholism as an emotional disorder and not a bad habit, are skeptical that demonstrating to alcoholics that the aftereffects of drinking are unpleasant (which many of them already know from bitter experience) is going to stop the process. What is needed, they say, is an emotional restructuring. Nevertheless, a growing number of studies indicate that loss of control over drinking does not inevitably follow one or two drinks (although it does seem to take over with more extensive drinking). With this knowledge, behavior modification techniques may become more widely accepted.

Alcoholism treatment has always been designed for men, with the few women who showed up handled as if they were merely smaller carbon copies. It is only recently that the special needs of women have been recognized. Although the disease may be the same, society's expectations give women added burdens and complicate their recovery. Researchers, finally looking at women who drink, have found to their surprise that, as one of them put it, "women are different." They have their own needs, reactions, and physiology. The shock has stimulated investigations into just how programs custom-made for men can be altered to fit the newly recognized female presence, as well as how special programs for women can be created.

There is a growing recognition that throughout the process of recovery—whether it takes place in a hospital, outpatient clinic, halfway house or doctor's office—women have special problems. Their needs include:

- Child-care facilities
- Treatment for double addiction
- An opportunity to recover in long-term living facilities which may be for women only
- Women's groups
- Treatment for lesbians
- Treatment for incest victims and battered women
- A choice of male or female counselors
- Insurance coverage to pay for long-term care

In addition, as Jonica D. Homiller suggested in her guidebook for state and local agencies, "Women of certain ethnic and cultural backgrounds (such as Chicano, Puerto Rican, Native American), in which the male 'macho' dominance is a deeply ingrained theme, will require unique consideration in that their communities are resistant to their seeking treatment. While their excessive drinking is seen as taboo, admitting it and coming forth for treatment are especially frowned upon."

Whatever their background, for alcoholic mothers a central question is, "Who will look after the children if I go into treatment?" Even getting to an appointment in an outpatient clinic can be a problem. The difficulties, of course, are often used as an excuse—or a reason—for not accepting or continuing treatment. But one clinic which had had trouble attracting women reports it is now crowded with patients because it set up a supervised playroom. It had found itself unexpectedly running an informal babysitting service in the hallway where mothers would take turns, and so decided to provide real child care.

For the mother who needs inpatient care, the problem is even more difficult. "If I had appendicitis I could ask my mother or a neighbor to take care of the kids, but I can't tell them I'm going into an alcoholic rehabilitation program," one woman said. A study of women referred to Meta House, a long-term residential facility in Milwaukee, showed that many decided against live-in treatment because there were young children at home. They felt too guilty to leave them. Sometimes this guilt becomes an excuse for avoiding treatment. A fortyish woman had started drinking heavily when her fifteen-year-old (the youngest) was out of the house a lot, and her husband was always working. She finally came into treatment in a Pennsylvania rehabilitation center that requires a thirty- to forty-day stay. Within two days, she had left. "I have to go home. My children need me," is what she said, forgetting she had come because she felt useless and unneeded.

There is another problem. Women are afraid that if they reveal themselves as alcoholic, their children will be taken away and put in foster care or in the custody of their fathers. "These fears have often been well founded," Dr. LeClair Bissell says, "so that women who have been sober and drug-free for years are still deprived of even minimal contact with their children." A middle-aged mother whose ex-husband had gained custody of their three teen-aged children says bitterly, "He never hesitated to leave the kids with me when I was drinking. Now that I'm in treatment, he's taken them away."

A pilot program to keep mothers and children together, at home, while treatment progressed, had its beginning in California. The University of California at Los Angeles trained paraprofessionals to go into the homes of alcoholic women and act as "surrogate mothers," making sure child care was adequate and lifting some of the practical burdens so the family could stay together. The program ended when federal funds were withdrawn.

Family House, in a working-class neighborhood just outside of Philadelphia, is one of the few places in the country where mothers and their children can stay together while the mother is treated. The rambling fourteen-room frame house with the wide porch looks like the home of any neighborhood family with a large brood of children. There are pint-sized tricycles outside and a sturdy fence to keep children from running into the road. Inside, women who have problems with alcohol and other drugs (most are also addicted to tranquilizers or amphetamines and even heroin) learn to understand themselves better, to prepare for school or a job, to run a household, and to be better parents. They live at Family House for six months to a year.

The mothers have ranged in age from eighteen to thirty. Some of these mothers have babies while they are in treatment, and they also become members of the household. Older children up to the age of ten go to local nursery schools or to the modern public elementary school just a block away. Florence Ershun, who was the director of Family House when it opened in 1975 with a grant from the NIAAA, says of her residents, "Almost all of them came from terrible backgrounds. Many of them have alcoholic parents. I'd say close to half have had incestuous relationships with their fathers or a brother. They are psychologically mixed-up people, just like their parents were. We're trying to break the cycle so their children won't be mixed up."

A senior counselor for eight women and twelve children living in the house is a young single mother herself, struggling to bring up a child on her own. She points out that the alcoholic woman escapes from her kids when she's drinking. "Then," she continues, "the alcohol isn't there, but the kids are. How is she going to cope with them, and with her guilt for neglecting them? We try to help her learn to be a good parent." They also try to help her stay sober: "We stress sobriety, but our major emphasis is on positive goals—achieve them, and sobriety will come along." Attendance at AA is encouraged, but not required—so is attendance at Parents Helping Parents, a self-help group for child abusers. The women are also referred to Planned Parenthood sessions. The residents polish their job skills and learn about nutrition and cooking by shopping for and preparing meals for the house.

In contrast to many other treatment facilities, Family House does not automatically dismiss a woman who has had a "slip"—gone back to drinking. "We decided," Carol Roman, the director, explains, "to operate on a no-fail basis. They're here for an alcohol or drug problem and if they demonstrate the symptoms of their illness, it's no reason to get rid of them. But if someone brings drugs or alcohol into the house, that's different. That threatens the whole community and can't be tolerated." Since most of the mothers drank heavily during their pregnancies, there are usually two children a year who exhibit the symptoms of the Fetal Alcohol Syndrome. "Most of our kids are very bright, though," Ms. Roman adds. "The one thing we have found consistently is that they tend to have low birth weights."

In follow-ups, 50 percent of the house's residents who completed the program were working or in school, had their children with them, and had all stayed sober. One of the successful graduates is now a secretary in the psychiatry department at Eagleville Hospital, parent facility of the halfway house. Her husband was a heroin addict; she had used the drug, too. By the time she and her five-year-old son came to live at the house she had given up heroin and was an alcoholic. She had tried to kill herself, landed in a hospital detoxification unit, and gone from there right to Family House. "I wouldn't have come into treatment if I couldn't have taken Jimmy along," she says. "There was nobody to take him." At the house she learned a lot about being a mother and how to do without alcohol. "I used to bark at Jimmy. I never hit him, but I gave him orders and expected him to jump. He was terrified of me, but now we're friends. I learned that at Family House. I understand that he has feelings, and we can talk to each other. He gets into his share of trouble now, but I don't treat him the same way. I've even learned to let him see his father."

Cathy and her son live within a few blocks of Family House, and Jimmy still sees his friends on the staff. This "staying close to home" is typical of women who go through the program. Many of them settle in the area and maintain the friendships they made while they lived in the halfway house. For some, it is the only family living they have known, and the staff and "graduates" have become an extended family network, people they can call on in time of need. Not only do the courts let the children live with their mothers despite the often damaging diagnosis of alcoholism, they have sometimes removed a child from a foster home and returned him to his mother because she was in the program.

Halfway houses have been a part of alcoholism treatment for a long time. They started when a recovered alcoholic would take another alcoholic home, feed him, house him, and help him get back on his feet. Many are still run by nonprofessionals who provide a place to live, AA involvement, and emotional support. Some of them are not really halfway steps back to the community; they are long-term care facilities for people who cannot make it in the outside world. In the days before alcoholism was recognized as a disease, they were called flophouses. Others offer a few months to a year of living in a protected environment, providing a bridge from the acute phase of treatment back into productive living. With the belated discovery that women, too, are alcoholic and there are some times they need to be separated from men, there are now about fifty halfway houses for women only in the country. There are almost 600 that accept men.

One of the first women-only facilities was Meta House, in Milwaukee. Francine Feinberg, its director, emphasizes the need for at least ninety days in a halfway house as a necessary part of treatment. Women need time to change. "When drugs and alcohol are taken away they are left with zero. The typical woman in treatment goes from alcohol to an eating disorder to a man. Here, we try to interrupt that cycle and teach people how to live. We help our younger women grow up and our older women grab onto the skills they used to have and develop new ones. And if a woman drank because of an inconsiderate husband (marital problems are high on the list of reasons) she can't go right back to the fighting or two or three kids clamoring for her attention." Ms. Feinberg, petite and youthful, calls herself "a relaxed role model" for the women she helps. She is not a recovering alcoholic herself although all the counselors in her program are. The facilities include a "three-quarter-way" house in a suburb to help ease the transition to independent living.

Meta House itself provides a serene setting with strict rules to help a woman stay away from alcohol and other drugs and begin to build a new life. Actually two trim frame houses on a quiet residential street, the emphasis here is on getting back into the world. There are fresh flowers on the dining room table and enticing smells in the kitchen. After a month of counseling, vocational testing, and a chance to catch her breath, a woman is encouraged to go out and find a job. Part-time, if that's all she can manage, or volunteer work, if, as some do, she feels guilty about taking a paid job when she doesn't need the money. Residents are mostly lower middle class, whose treatment is paid for by public funds and private contributions that help support the house. Once they start working, they contribute toward their own care.

It is a drug-free environment (except for doctor-prescribed antipsychotics and antidepressants)—even aspirin is kept locked up and dispensed only by staff members. A woman who drinks or takes pills may be given one more chance, but the pervasive atmosphere is one of abstinence. Some women cannot tolerate the demands. Newcomers still struggle with their desire to drink. "I really like Scotch," one recalled dreamily. "And two or three martinis and you really feel mellow. It helps," she says, coming back to reality, "to have the rules and restrictions. I know if I break them I'll be back where I started from. The rules act as a deterrent." Like so many other women, she was addicted to tranquilizers, too. "And I still feel pretty jumpy sometimes. They say it takes six months really to get the stuff out of your system."

At April House, too, many of the women have drug addictions. Opened in Milwaukee in the late 1970s, April House is a halfway house for women who are indigent; some of them have no family or friends. They live in a yellow brick building that used to be a Jewish home for the aged, and join men alcoholics next door for group therapy as well as activity and work therapies. It is, unlike Meta House, a facility for women that has a close relationship with one for men. And, with its echoing corridors, it has an institutional feel.

These houses operate at about 80 percent capacity because, says Bishop Walter X. Brown, director of both facilities, "In order to get public funding, there has to be prior approval for each individual. This means that those who really need the services can get them, and those who don't really work at changing themselves are no longer taking up those beds."

Government requirements often affect treatment. Fund-granting agencies may insist that certain medical standards be met that are beyond the reach of some halfway houses, traditionally run by former alcoholics. Time limits (insurance coverage may end in ninety days) may also force people back into the community before they're ready.

For the women who do come into April House, there are the usual group and individual counseling, the opportunity to practice vocational skills in a sheltered workshop, and a chance to work on their pictures of themselves. A major problem, as it is every place, is low self-esteem. Edith, a gray-haired woman in flowered smock and slacks who looks older than her fifty years, summed up the feelings of most recovering alcoholic women when she lowered her head during an interview and murmured, "I'm so ashamed. I'm so ashamed."

In her three months at April House, though, Edith has begun to appreciate what life can be like when you're sober. "The best thing is I'm starting to notice things again and everything is so beautiful. When I was drinking, I didn't see anything. I was in another world. Now I don't miss a thing."

In her women's group, Edith is beginning to respect herself and develop her own individuality. This, says Francine Feinberg of Meta House, is one of the reasons for putting women in their own groups. Another is to give them an opportunity to explore their sexuality and their relationships with men. "These women," she points out, "seem to be very giving. Unfortunately, they have been giving and have been taken advantage of. They have to learn to trust other women and not fall into the same 'pleasing' pattern with men. For some, Meta House is the first place they've ever had close relationships with women, and they learn there's a whole new world of support." Meta House often has one male counselor; what he does is provide a "safe" male to learn to love. He won't take advantage of the women, as other men have, and he can help them move on to healthier relationships in the future.

This problem with men is a pervasive one. At Rockland Psychiatric Center in New York State, the women's group tackles these loaded areas. One counselor, herself a recovered alcoholic, says, "Many of us feel that our worth has to be reckoned in the coin of the realm—being somehow attached to a male. We expect to be taken care of, and so the competition gets pretty keen, woman against woman. We try to open up the tremendous resource of other women who can be encouraging and nurturing instead of the stereotype of two-faced and double-dealing."

Women also feel freer to discuss their sexual experiences and attitudes out of earshot of men. An attractive group participant admits, "I could never talk about the way I picked up men in a bar when I was drinking if there were men around. I'd be too embarrassed." Unlike this woman, many alcoholic women report diminished sex drives, and studies on sex-role confusion hint that the promiscuity seen in a small proportion may be an attempt to prove their femininity to themselves—as well as a way to pay for drinking. Frigidity is reported more often than the popular fantasy of sexual abandon.

These for-women-only treatment and recovery groups can also help women work on problems that are not directly related to alcohol use. Some have felt that AA is not geared to this broader picture, and that they need another or a supplementary group in which to work things out. Leona Kent of the San Mateo, California, Women's Rehabilitation Association pointed out, "AA has not been dealing with the problems of depression that remain after you've recovered. When my husband died I wanted to go right back to the bottle. I couldn't find anyone at AA who would listen to my problems. If I told them that I was on the verge of having another drink they would all be there helping me. But no one wanted to share my grief over my husband."

Another woman who feels gaps in the AA program is Dr. Jean Kirkpatrick, a founder of Women for Sobriety, in Quakertown, Pennsylvania, a nonprofit organization with 200 groups in thirty-five states, Canada, Australia, New Zealand, and Iceland. Women for Sobriety reaches out to the kinds of women who are not touched by traditional programs until very late. "One of the things about alcoholism is that it creeps up," she explains. "The woman alone comes home to an empty apartment. She has one drink, then two, then three and then goes without dinner. I'm talking about the woman who in the past has not gotten help until she was carried out to a hospital. We are reaching the wives of executives and the professional women who live alone."

This program of women helping women also offers more privacy than large AA meetings. "If they go to these meetings, they're afraid they'll meet too many people they know," a suburban group leader points out. "They're scared. Many of them are still drinking and trying to find out how severe their problem is. So they start by meeting in private homes."

Women for Sobriety offers a positive approach with thirteen steps to recovery. These include "I am what I think," "Negative emotions destroy only myself," and "Happiness is a habit I will develop." Consciousness raising is also part of the program, but a group leader (herself a recovered alcoholic) emphasized, "There's no magic potion. No consciousness raising can stop a woman's drinking. First she has to stop drinking, then she can work on her personality." Many of the women who participate also attend AA meetings for the extra support, but they find they can talk about particularly feminine concerns with more ease in their small at-home groups.

All these therapies, designed especially for women or used to treat all alcoholics, have some success, but none are strikingly more successful than others. As psychiatrist Donald Goodwin laments, "There is no penicillin for alcoholism." Many treatment approaches are used in combination, throwing the whole therapeutic weaponry against the defiant disease. Obviously, in a condition as complex as alcoholism, nothing is going to work for everyone, and the factors that contribute to success seem to have very little to do with what kind of treatment was offered. As a matter of fact, Dr. Edith Gomberg of the University of Michigan insists, "In a deviance disorder like alcoholism, the attitude (conscious and unconscious) of the therapist toward women and toward alcoholism and the enthusiasm and interest of the therapist seem far more related to outcome than the techniques used." Supporting this viewpoint is the fact that the one study showing much higher rates of success with women than with men was conducted by two experienced women therapists, Vernelle Fox and M. A. Smith.

Another humbling reality emerged when D. A. Thomas compared ninety successful patients with ninety unsuccessful patients. The women who did not make it were more likely to have fathers who were alcoholic, more likely to be double addicted, and had more physical illnesses because of drinking. The successful women had changed their friends; they now spent more time with people who drank little, and they had better relationships with their families. In another study conducted by J. H. Glover and P. A. McCue there were more successes in women over forty who had stable marriages—whether they had been given "talking" therapies or subjected to electric shock aversion made no difference.

Whether older or younger women have a better chance of recovery is debatable; there are statistics to buttress either attitude. But workers in the field have been noticing that women in treatment have been getting younger, and that women who start problem drinking early in life are generally harder to treat. As one study pointed out, they have few incentives to stop drinking. "[They] have never had very much and have little hope of getting more [so] they drink to escape that devastating reality. . . ." But treatment at a younger age may also mean that the woman started drinking later, has been drinking fewer years, and has come for help early in the disease process. She stands a better chance of success.

This conclusion was part of a look at eighty studies of treatment successes and failures in eight countries. Three American researchers, headed by Dr. Raymond M. Costello of the University of Texas, concluded that the programs with the best track records (without distinguishing between men and women) had three things in common: They carefully selected their patients instead of attempting the gargantuan task of treating large numbers of diverse alcoholics; they used Antabuse enthusiastically; and they offered a wide range of therapeutic services, from individual sessions to family therapy to job finding. In addition, "The incentive to retain or regain through abstinence what one has lost or might lose because of drinking can be a powerful therapeutic ally." Without the clear belief that life will get worse if drinking continues, and much better if it stops, the chances for success are slim.

Finally, a study of women at a state alcoholic rehabilitation center showed that even with low educational achievement and occupational status, the women who did best were the ones with the highest intelligence.[4] What seems to matter most, then, is not whether a woman is given psychotherapy or behavior therapy or inpatient care as against outpatient care, or is in women's groups as against mixed groups. What counts very largely is who the patient is. If she still has her health, a stable family, and good intellectual abilities, she is more likely to recover.

But it is risky to try to make predictions about individual lives on the basis of statistics. "There are always extreme cases where you have doubt about the outcome," says one alcoholism counselor who wasted years in drinking, "but I happen to be an eternal optimist, and for myself I believe recovery is a gift—a grace. Many times if someone had looked at me, they'd have thought I wouldn't make it."

How to define "making it" is another problem. Most surveys use sobriety as the yardstick; there is just beginning to be a recognition that this may not be the whole answer. Some alcoholics who remain sober continue to have social, economic, and family problems. Harold Conlow, when director of the chemical dependency unit at St. Vincent's Hospital in Sioux City, Iowa, warned, "Often her male companions drink heavily even though she no longer does. This can sometimes frustrate a man to the point where he may beat the woman or even kill her." In addition, Dr. Asbjorn Medhus, in a follow-up study of eighty-three "skid-row" alcoholic women in Sweden, found they died of accidents or suicide at alarming rates within ten years of their first compulsory treatment. Their accidental death rate was seventy times higher than the general population; they were thirty times more likely to kill themselves. Many of them were drinking despite treatment, and they were clearly a multi-problem population. But their high mortality, even when sober, emphasizes the reality that rehabilitation evidently involves more than just freedom from alcohol.

An American who runs a comprehensive alcoholism treatment center for men and women in London says, "Recovery is about living a normal life. Minimal success is people being dry and functioning. Maximum success is when they're living comfortable lives up to their potentials, in which drink has ceased to bug them."

Even after the alcoholic is sober, she may have trouble reestablishing a normal life because of the stigma of her illness. A New York City survey revealed a "dramatic denial of rights" for recovered alcoholics, "not only in employment, but in welfare, insurance and child custody." Allan Luks, head of the New York City affiliate of the National Council on Alcoholism, told this story at a hearing on discrimination against recovered alcoholics: "A female with five years' sobriety applied for a job with the Police Department and, after informing them of her past drinking problems, was rejected. She filed suit and won the court battle." New York City has now passed the first ordinance in the country prohibiting discrimination in jobs, education, and housing for recovered alcoholics.

Child custody is still a problem. Dr. LeClair Bissell tells of women whose children had been placed in foster homes and who were unable to reclaim them even after treatment. "In alcoholism," she says, "I know of no legal definition of recovery."

Most agencies consider abstinence to be recovery. The National Council on Alcoholism reports that 98 percent of people who have been sober for two years never return to chronic drinking. The NIAAA estimates that 50–75 percent of alcoholics still married and living at home who get treatment can be counted as successes—they are able to keep a job, maintain their marriages, and continue to be respected members of their communities. For some, less fortunate in the social and community supports to which they can return, treatment becomes a revolving door. There is a widely used figure (based on AA estimates) that 50 percent of women return to drinking within six weeks of inpatient treatment.

More than 60 percent are repeaters in all types of alcoholism services. These figures have to be looked at with caution. All alcoholic populations contain hard-core drinkers who seem to be untouched by therapeutic efforts. These are the men and women who use inpatient services for "three hots and a bed" as they used to use police lockups, and they distort the figures on recovery and return. Industrial programs which reach people earlier, while they are still functioning well, have much better results. E. I. duPont de Nemours, which has had an alcoholism program since 1942, has a combined man-woman success rate of 80 percent. Other companies report about 70 percent. How this applies to women is hard to determine—they tend to avoid treatment by moving to another job or just staying home to drink. "Go into treatment or you lose your job"—the reality therapy that makes industrial programs notably successful—doesn't have the same force for women.

Are women sicker than men and harder to treat? It is possible to find studies that say yes and those that say no. That women alcoholics are seen as worse than men may play a part in keeping them out of treatment until they are carried into a hospital; at that point, there is no question they are "sicker" than most of the men. Certainly it is true that women alcoholics more often have diagnosed mental disorders. But, as Dr. Marc Schuckit points out in his book, *Alcoholism Problems in Women and Children*, "The interpretation of the higher degree of psychological dysfunction in women alcoholics is unclear: Does alcoholism cause more psychiatric disorder in women? *or* does a woman have to be more 'ill' to overcome the more intense social stigma against heavy drinking and demonstrated alcoholism? *or* do women displaying alcoholism more frequently have other major psychiatric disorders of which alcohol problems are symptomatic? *or* is psychiatric disorder in women alcoholics the result of the severe social sanctions taken against women who abuse alcohol?" No one knows the answers yet. But the impression over the years has been that women are harder to engage in treatment, leave more quickly, and are more difficult to manage. Winnie Fraser, director of a Canadian detoxification unit, observed, 'Women generally present many more management difficulties than do the men, during both their admission and their stay. They are usually more deteriorated than men, physically and emotionally, and more abrasive, more aggressive, and perhaps also more manipulative. While they take longer to detoxify than men, they do not stay as long and are much less willing to be engaged in further treatment." This reluctance to stay in treatment may be based on several things: family pressure and guilt ("The children need me"), the psychological isolation of women alcoholics which makes them difficult to reach, and perhaps the fact that they may use treatment facilities differently.

The painful loneliness of the woman drinker became poignantly evident in a study of drinking behavior done by D. A. Tracey and Peter E. Nathan, psychologists at Rutgers University. Four alcoholic women—all still living in intact families—were daily drinkers who saved their drinking until their household tasks were done. In the hospital, they earned "points" to spend for either alcohol or the company of others. They chose socialization. "The solitary female drinker portrayed by writers in the field may reflect social sanctions against women frequenting bars alone rather than a preference for seclusion," the study concluded. The fact remains that women are more likely to be loners and less likely to become attached to others in the treatment program in a way that holds them. "Women" said Ms. Fraser, "tend to isolate themselves and are much more difficult to engage in discussion."

On the other hand, a survey of outpatient treatment programs in New York State found a lower dropout rate for women—partly because they are inclined to "talk out" rather than "act out" their problems, and partly because the women in these programs were younger and seemed more stable than the men. The agencies which did report a higher dropout rate for females cited the universally recognized problems of low self-esteem and lack of childcare facilities.

A better understanding of what kind of person sticks it out can come from a look at men who were given a series of Rorschach and other psychological tests. The ones who remained in treatment were more intelligent, loyal, persistent, verbal, anxious, and dissatisfied with themselves. The dropouts were restless, impulsive, less dependable, and less inhibited by anxiety.[5]

But the in-again, out-again pattern that many women have may not indicate a lack of success. In a follow-up study at a rural state hospital, researcher B. J. Fitzgerald found that "a higher dropout rate among women can be anticipated during their first treatment attempt. However, this dropout rate does not appear to have the same significance as in men. While in men, noncompletion on first admission is a rough predictor of noncompletion in a second treatment attempt, for women this predictor cannot be used as effectively. Many of the women who are good prospects for later treatment efforts drop out of the program during their first try."

There are other optimistic findings. Recent preliminary studies of middle-class women in private hospital treatment (in contrast to the largely public-facility population studied before) indicate that women may have slightly higher success rates than men. Found earlier and treated with recognition of their special needs, they get better as fast, or faster.

Many therapists from a cross section of professional disciplines still find recovery rates from alcoholism distressingly low. This has led recently to a questioning of the traditional approaches.

Since it is so difficult to keep people in treatment, is long-term treatment really necessary or particularly effective? A study at the Family Alcoholism Clinic of the Institute of Psychiatry in London suggests that it might not be. Fifty married male alcoholics were given one long psychiatric interview with their wives; fifty others, matched for age, marital status, etc., went through the traditional treatment program: counseling, medication, AA meetings, and psychotherapy. There were no significant differences in treatment outcome for the two groups in a two-year follow-up. Dr. Jim Orford, one of the researchers, says, "The conclusion we came to was that there is more scope than people have previously thought for fairly brief counseling. Our treatment in the single interview consisted of not assuming the people had a knowledge of their problem, but giving them a clear idea of what was wrong and a clear idea of what they should do about it. Too often people who drink get confusing advice. One person says 'Stop drinking' and the other person says, 'Oh, nonsense. You don't drink anymore than I do.' "

In the one-interview approach, the patient was given a clear idea of what further drinking was likely to do to him and told quite simply and plainly to stop. The responsibility for change was clearly up to the man and his family. With this approach, many of them did stop—about as many as stopped after much longer treatment. The results, though, may not be that clear-cut because in both cases there was long-term contact. Even in the "advice" group, a social worker visited the wife once a month for the first year. And the researchers caution, "it must remain an open question whether similar results would be found with a series of women alcoholics."

Since 50–75 percent drop out after only a few interviews in the majority of clinics, a one-interview technique might make it possible to reach many more people successfully. This isn't the only study to suggest that there may be alternatives to the long-term traditional approaches. After five years of experience with almost five thousand patients, the Cleveland Center on Alcoholism[6] found that many could be helped by as few as one to five sessions. Clearly, a review of treatment strategies is in order.

Another even more emotion-laden reappraisal is now taking place. The orthodox view has been "once an alcoholic, always an alcoholic." There is no cure, only management. Treatment programs (except a few using behavior modification) have all been aimed at total abstinence—"one drink, and you will progress inevitably to chronic alcoholism" has been the message. But two studies of more than one thousand alcoholics released in 1976 and 1980 by the Rand Corporation, a Santa Monica, California, think-tank, suggested that some could indeed return safely to social drinking. The researchers warned that they were not suggesting that recovered alcoholics test themselves by drinking; only that there seemed to be some people who, not able to achieve abstinence, did not inevitably become drunk.

The alcoholics in the study were in treatment at a center supported by NIAAA; only men were included in the final analysis. The women, the report said, drank so much less than the men that they would have distorted the statistical analysis. Besides, there were too few women and since there is "substantial evidence that alcoholism is much more prevalent among men, we do not feel these exclusions represent serious limitations." Once again, the fact that proportionally fewer women come into treatment has justified the pretense that they don't exist. The first report created a furor. It was criticized for its criteria and its statistics, for being poorly done (follow-ups were only six months and eighteen months after treatment), and for overlooking the possibility that these people were in "spontaneous remission." There are many diseases—cancer among them—in which people recover inexplicably, and alcoholism may be one of these. Dr. Morris Chafetz did not share the panic of many of his colleagues: "The Rand study was the sixtieth to confirm findings that, for reasons we don't understand, a small percentage of severe alcoholics can go back to social drinking. There have since been two more studies confirming this. They are interesting research findings, but I don't know anyone who recommends research findings as treatment goals. They obviously don't apply to everyone, and can be dangerously wrong for some."

One of the studies that turned up problem drinkers who could drink moderately was a community mental-health survey in 1960–61 in the Washington Heights section of New York City. To the surprise of the researchers, some people who had been problem drinkers reported they were now able to keep their drinking within acceptable limits. Social workers Margaret Bailey and Jean Stewart followed up on these people five years later. One of them was a young woman whose parents had both been alcoholic. Her heavy drinking began after her engagement was broken and her mother offered her a drink "to make her feel better." She started drinking to unconsciousness every night, having blackouts, and drinking her way through weekends. The change came after she married and moved out of her parents' house. She "saw the parallel between my own and my mother's drinking," and was able to cut down to two to four beers a day. At the time of the last interview she was pregnant for the second time and had been able to stick to moderate drinking for seven years.

When Drs. Marc Schuckit and George Winokur looked at forty-five women alcoholics three years after they had been admitted to treatment in St. Louis hospitals, they stumbled on a surprising eleven women who were able to drink socially. The doctors caution that this was a small sample and that further research is needed, but it may indicate that "a substantial percent of some groups of women alcoholics can return to social drinking."

Dr. Sheila Blume suggests that those who were able to moderate their drinking in all these surveys accomplished this only because they were really aiming for abstinence. She may be right. A study of the subtle effects of social influence on drinking patterns confirmed that praising the goal of abstinence was more helpful in reducing drinking than supporting the idea that taking a drink or two couldn't hurt.[7] As Dr. Blume warns, "many alcoholics drink moderately for a while, then, if not interrupted, will escalate their drinking."

The emotional reaction to the idea that some alcoholics may be able to resume normal drinking can be understood, according to Dr. Ron Roizen of the School of Public Health at the University of California, if we realize that "from a traditionalist's standpoint, an attack on the abstinence criterion is an attack on the classical disease concept of alcoholism. And undercutting that truth is only done at great peril because embracing that truth proves to be the most successful treatment known for the condition." It is important, he suggests, to separate utility (it works) from validity (it is based on correct assumptions).

Certainly controlled drinking has been demonstrated many times in hospital settings—some of them outfitted to resemble bars, with dim lights, music, and an understanding bartender. Follow-up studies have also shown that the social drinking pattern was sometimes maintained. After researching the literature on abstinence versus controlled drinking, psychologists William R. Miller and Glenn R. Caddy concluded: "Both abstinence and controlled drinking therapies are now needed." For the alcoholic with physical damage, of course, abstinence is the only answer, but for others the treatment establishment is, after long reluctance, finally beginning to look at broader possibilities. Eagleville Hospital and Rehabilitation Center in Pennsylvania began a conference on the problem with this explanation: "We have been aware, for instance, that recovered staff persons are using marijuana or engaging in social drinking while demanding total abstinence from their clients. This has led us to at least investigate the possibilities of less than total abstinence for recovered persons." However, by the end of the conference, the participants concluded "total abstinence is the treatment objective for all our programs."

To his fellow physicians who are so protective of the abstinence concept that they refuse to look at new findings, Dr. Eric W. Fine wrote in a letter in the *Journal of the American Medical Association* that "the alcoholic population consists of several subgroups with different etiologies, clinical manifestations, natural histories, and outcomes. They therefore demand—and deserve—different treatment approaches based on carefully determined individualized treatment approaches." He adds that patients who have not responded to the abstinence approach, as well as younger men and women, diagnosed early, who are unwilling to face a long life without alcohol, might benefit from this new attitude. Yet a study (reported in the *New England Journal of Medicine* for June 27,

1985) that followed more than a thousand people for five to seven years after they had been treated for alcoholism found that fewer than 2 percent were able to drink socially. "This study suggests," the researchers concluded, "that there is little cause for optimism about the likelihood of an evolution to long-term, stable, moderate drinking among treated alcoholics." Abstinence, they said, is the only feasible approach.

Nobody knows why one person loses control of drinking and another doesn't, and there is not yet any way to winnow out those few alcoholics who might—and those who can't—safely resume the use of alcohol. Until some sort of sensitivity test is developed, the sanest treatment is, of course, the time-honored one. As research continues, however, it may be possible to identify individuals who are problem drinkers yet can be helped to modify, and not necessarily end, their drinking.

11

A Guide to Sensible Drinking

A drink or two releases inhibitions, makes strangers like each other, and adds an indefinable ambience to good food and good friends. But three-quarters of all drinkers surveyed recently said they thought alcohol did more harm than good. In the face of this ambivalence we go on drinking, hoping to find the perfect way to enjoy the pleasures and avoid the consequences of this legendary social lubricant.

Some enlightenment can come from the results of research already considered in this book. Based on what is now known, here are some practical tips for pleasurable drinking:

Know Your Drinks

Sensible drinking depends on understanding how much alcohol is in what kind of drink, and what happens when the drink hits bottom. The startling truth is a six-pack of beer has as much alcohol as six highballs, or six glasses of wine.

Liquor facts at a glance:

"Proof" equals twice the alcohol content. 80-proof liquor is 40 percent alcohol.

A shot of whiskey (one and one-half ounces), a bottle of beer, and a four-ounce glass of wine have the same alcohol content. As one expert emphasized, "A drink is a drink is a drink."

Hard liquor is usually 40 percent alcohol by volume, wine up to 14 percent, and domestic beer 6 percent (imported beers tend to be stronger). The quantities consumed in a standard "drink," though, make them equivalent.

Ladylike drinkers of sherry should be aware that its alcohol content is fortified—to about 20 percent. Liqueurs and cordials have about 40 percent—the same as hard liquor.

The cereal in beer may slow down the absorption of alcohol from the stomach into the bloodstream and so may tomato juice or fruit juices in some mixed drinks. Thirty to sixty minutes after starting a drink you are likely to feel the maximum effect.

The stomach, when irritated, has an automatic shutoff valve which may keep undiluted liquor from passing quickly into the intestines. That's why a slug of Scotch in a sensitive stomach may be absorbed slowly and have less of an intoxicating effect than a glass of wine. It will, though, assail the stomach and may even cause tissue to slough off.

A cold shower, exercise, or a pot of coffee won't speed the process of sobering up. The only thing known that makes the body burn alcohol faster than about one drink an hour is fructose—fruit sugar—in massive, sickening doses.

Don't Mix Alcohol with Certain Medications

Newspaper columnist Dorothy Kilgallen combined sleeping pills and a few drinks and was found dead in bed the next morning—an "accidental suicide." Karen Ann Quinlan, the young woman whose coma started an investigation into the use of machines to sustain life, was evidently also a victim of this often lethal combination. There are other things, too, that shouldn't be taken with alcohol, and since doctors prescribe much more often for women than for men, it's important that women understand what the possible consequences are. Researcher Muriel Nellis estimates that seventy million women run into trouble adding alcohol to pills.

Barbiturates-Seconal. This is like adding a "downer" to a "downer" and the results can be fatal.

Minor tranquilizers—Valium, Librium. Each pill is like adding another drink or, some researchers feel, even more than just one. It was this kind of combination that evidently put former first lady Betty Ford into the hospital.

Anti-depressants—Endep, Sinequan, Triavil. Particularly for the menopausal woman, it's important to understand that these drugs also multiply the effects of alcohol. The result is likely to be slurred speech and unsteady gait.

Flagyl. This is used to treat the common vaginal infection caused by monilia. In combination with alcohol it can cause headache and nausea.

Learn to Recognize Your Own Body Cues

Judith Seixas, a psychologist specializing in alcohol-abuse prevention, suggests that if you know your mind starts to get fuzzy or you feel sick when you've had enough, stop. Other experts point out that there are easily noticeable results of drinking: first, a feeling of warmth and slight numbness in the cheeks and lips; then, tingling in the hands, arms, and legs; and eventually a hint of numbness in the extremities. When fingers and toes start reacting it means the blood-alcohol level is probably approaching 0.1—the usual legal limit of intoxication. A person will feel higher on the rising curve—when she's getting high—than on the descending one, although blood-alcohol levels may be the same. What this means is that someone may insist, "I'm not high—I can drive," when, as a matter of fact, a breathalizer test will indicate intoxication.

If You Have More Than One Drink, Don't Drive

Studies have shown that the experienced driver is no more likely to have an accident after one drink than after none. But after two drinks she is 50 percent more likely to get into trouble on the road. Not that she is legally drunk—it's just that she's convinced she can drive better, although her ability to judge speed and distance has been impaired. What Dr. E. M. Jellinek, dean of alcohol researchers at Yale, used to recommend is this: If you take two ounces of whiskey, wait about one hour before you drive. If it's four ounces, wait two hours—and for each extra ounce add an extra hour.

The new driver had better stay away from liquor completely; recently learned skills are the first to dissolve in alcohol.

Give Your Body a Fighting Chance

Avoid "down the hatch" situations or Russian-style vodka toasts. Undiluted, concentrated spirits jolt the brain and damage delicate membranes. White wine is preferable to red—particularly French red wines—because the reds are likely to contain tannin, identified as being associated with some kinds of stomach cancer. If you're a regular drinker, give your body time to recover. A dry day or two in among the wet ones will prolong the health of your liver and the strength of your muscles. And the regular drinker who reaches four drinks a day had better cut down, even though she's functioning well. The National Council on Alcoholism reports that the heavy drinker increases astronomically her chances of becoming alcoholic.

There's no question that the safest way to drink is to sip wine or beer with meals.

Don't Drink Water Before You Drink Alcohol

Although water is fine to dilute liquor, water in an empty stomach will speed the absorption of alcohol and tend to make you drunk faster.

Watch Out for Bubbles

Carbonated mixers, such as soda and ginger ale, send the alcohol into your bloodstream faster. That's why champagne produces a fast high—the carbonation, not the alcohol content, makes the difference.

Eat Before You Drink or With Your Drinks

A full stomach retards the rate at which alcohol is absorbed and acts as a buffer between liquor and delicate mucous membranes. Although a drink may go down smoothly, when it hits bottom it acts like sandpaper, irritating the areas it touches directly. It is this irritation that produces heartburn and stomach upset.

There's a lot of conflicting folklore about what to eat before or with a drink. Dr. Henry B. Murphree of Rutgers University has suggested fatty proteins—cheese and dairy products, for instance—because these tend to blot up the alcohol and stay around longer. The Russians swear by caviar, and some people insist a slug of olive oil produces an impervious lining. But Dr. Jack H. Mendelson of the National Institute of Mental Health surveyed the often controversial results of research on the effects of food and ethanol absorption and says remorselessly, "None of these data supports popular folklore that a specific food (e.g., milk) has a unique effect in reducing ethanol absorption." What seems to matter though is that food—evidently any food—in the stomach will slow things down.

When Dieting, Match Your Drinking to Your Waistline

Since alcohol's effect is closely tied to body weight, someone who loses twenty pounds will get high faster than she used to. There's another problem with liquor and dieting. One of the first effects of a drink is to release inhibition and stimulate the appetite. Weight Watchers, for instance, says "no" to alcohol because it makes it harder to say "no" to food. Alcohol is also just empty calories—about one hundred in an ounce of 100-proof liquor.

A recent study by Canadian researcher J. Murray McLaughlan found that a person may become dangerously drunk on only two or three drinks after dieting for a few days. Restricting carbohydrates (as most diets do) lowers blood sugar; so, evidently, does alcohol. Exercise lowers it even more. The combination can produce what looks like drunkenness, even though blood-alcohol levels aren't high. The dizziness and stumbling are really symptoms of hypoglycemia.

Keep an Eye on Your Menstrual Cycle

Just before your period begins, according to University of Oklahoma researchers, you're apt to get your maximum reaction to drink. On the day the flow starts, the effect is at its lowest. In the middle of the menstrual cycle the blood-alcohol level falls somewhere between the high and low points. Because of this variation, Dr. Ben M. Jones points out, "A woman may not feel very intoxicated on two drinks in the middle of her menstrual cycle, but may become very intoxicated on two drinks at the end of her menstrual cycle [just before her period begins]." Being aware can help you adjust your drinking to your hormonal levels.

If You're Pregnant, Don't Drink

Not all the evidence is in yet, but it seems silly to take unnecessary chances where the health and development of an infant are concerned. Although some doctors still recommend a drink now and then to ease digestion and calm discomfort, no one yet knows exactly what effect even small doses of alcohol may have on a developing fetus. It seems safest, too, for a nursing mother to avoid drinking; the alcohol passes quickly into her milk.

If You're Sick, Don't Drink

Liquor has an abrasive effect on tender tissues. Even though it may temporarily ease the pain of a sore throat or an upset stomach, it won't help the condition and may make things worse. When Wisconsin family physician Richard W. Shropshire studied the drinking habits of his patients, he found that two to six drinks a day produced or complicated physical complaints ranging from headaches to diarrhea to high blood pressure and insomnia. Anyone with a urinary-tract infection should also avoid the irritating effects of drinking. Other doctors add that using alcohol as a drug to treat illness may make you more likely to become addicted to it.

Going against current medical emphasis on danger, Dr. Morris Chafetz stresses the times alcohol does help: It can, he says, clear a stuffy nose by dilating the nasal passages. And it can anesthetize discomfort so the patient rests more easily. The message seems to be, as it is in so many cases with this chameleonlike substance, if you think it helps, it will. But use it in small quantities, and if things get worse, stop.

Try Not to Anticipate a Hangover

Its severity may have more to do with expectation than with intake, but there are things you can do to minimize it. Dr. Chafetz says the way you feel the morning after has a lot to do with the way you were feeling the night before. Alcohol dims sensations of fatigue and tension and lets you push beyond your limits. The next day the exhaustion hits and is labeled a hangover.

He realizes, of course, that this observation will probably rate highest on the list of things to ignore; the lift over that slump is one of the chief reasons for taking a drink.

The congeners in whatever you drink—substances other than alcohol that are produced or introduced during processing—may also add to your discomfort. These include the herbs of vermouth and the resins that seep in from barrels in which bourbon has been aged. Distilled spirits tend to have fewer of these toxic extras than wine; and vodka, particularly if it has been charcoal filtered, has fewest of all. This reputation for being hangover-free may account for its current top sales position in this country.

Mixing drinks won't make you sicker unless, of course, you're convinced that it will, and sauerkraut juice or a raw egg won't make you better unless, of course, you think they will. Sleep is the best remedy, and a few aspirin may help kill the headache.

Feel Free to Say "No."

If it's a day when you don't feel like the ritual drink before a business lunch or a cocktail before dinner, how can you avoid alcohol without putting a damper on other people's enjoyment? It's possible to be unobtrusive by sipping ginger ale and ice cubes or a Virgin Mary (tomato juice without the vodka). It's also possible to say, "No thanks, I don't like what it does to me," or "It's not good for me," without sounding like a moralist.

It's important to listen to your body cues. If you ordinarily drink but don't feel like it just then, you may be coming down with something. If you're feeling low, beware of heavy drinking—alcohol is a depressant. It should also be avoided before and during flying if you have a cold or tend to have ear problems. You may also be a person whose genetic makeup reacts to alcohol with a headache or flushing, or someone with a medical condition that makes it unwise. Whatever the reason, don't let yourself succumb to pressure by convention or the current social climate.

Be a Considerate Hostess

Craig Claiborne, the *New York Times* master of foods, sounded off on the dangers of a prolonged cocktail hour: "Woe be unto the host or hostess who schedules dinner at eight and sits me down (or props me up) for dinner at midnight." There's no virtue, either, in mixing extra stiff drinks "to get things started," in pushing refills during the evening, or in offering guests "one more for the road." It's a far better idea to have coffee and something to go with it at the evening's finish—not that coffee will sober anyone up (it won't), but time spent without liquor gives the body a breather and allows some of the alcohol to metabolize. You might even try to stop serving drinks an hour before the party is likely to end. For nondrinking friends, whatever their reason, the considerate hostess keeps soft drinks and fruit juice on hand and offers them as acceptable alternatives.

No one is saying never take a drink. And no one is pushing women to give up their ice cubes and ginger ale and start drinking liquor if they don't want to. What the experts keep trying to get across is the fact that alcohol can be a dangerous pleasure. The tricky thing about it is that it works; it is the world's oldest tranquilizer and should be treated with respect. Knowing its effects— good and bad—can help women cope with pressures that seem to equate social equality with social drinking.

Where to Write for Information and Pamphlets about Alcohol Use and Abuse

Addiction Research Foundation (ARF)
33 Russell Street
Toronto, Ontario
Canada M5S 2S1

ARF, a leading research center, also publishes books and pamphlets.

Alcohol and Drug Problems Association of North America
444 North Capitol Street, N.W.
Washington, D.C. 20001

National Clearinghouse for Alcohol Information (NCALI)
PO Box 2345
Rockville, Maryland 20852

NCALI provides annotated bibliographies, divided into subject areas; an information and education package on women and alcohol; and a package designed to help communities develop action programs.

National Council on Alcoholism Office on Prevention and
Education
12 West 21st Street
New York, New York 10010

This office has specific information about women's programs, plus a list of state task forces, many of which provide speakers as well as information about local programs.

National Institute on Alcohol Abuse and Alcoholism
5600 Fishers Lane
Rockville, Maryland 20852

12

Alcoholism Checklist and Resource Information

*T*here are a lot of checklists of danger signals—most of them based on what is known about men drinkers. One of the few aimed specifically at women was distributed by the Kansas City National Council on Alcoholism:*

To the Ladies

Are You an Alcoholic?

1. Do you try to get someone to buy liquor for you because you are ashamed to buy it yourself?
2. Do you buy liquor at different places so no one will know how much you purchase?
3. Do you hide the empties and dispose of them secretly?
4. Do you plan in advance to "reward" yourself with a little drinking bout after you've worked very hard in the house?
5. Are you often permissive with your children because you feel guilty about the way you behaved when you were drinking?

* Reprinted with permission. Jane James, Director, TAFWA Center, 3718 Tracy, Kansas City, Missouri 64109. Doris Saxon, Alcoholism Counselor, Johnson County Mental Health Center, 6000 Lamar, Shawnee Mission, Kansas.

6. Do you have "blackouts"—periods about which you remember nothing?

7. Do you ever phone the hostess of a party the next day and ask if you hurt anyone's feelings or made a fool of yourself?

8. Do you find cigarette holes in your clothes or the furniture and can't remember when it happened?

9. Do you take an extra drink or two before leaving for a party when you know liquor will be served there?

10. Do you often wonder if anyone knows how much you drink?

11. Do you feel wittier or more charming when you are drinking?

12. Do you feel panicky when faced with nondrinking days, such as a visit to out-of-town relatives?

13. Do you invent social occasions for drinking, such as inviting friends for lunch, cocktails, or dinner?

14. When others are present, do you avoid reading articles or seeing movies or TV shows about women alcoholics but read and watch when no one is around?

15. Do you ever carry liquor in your purse?

16. Do you become defensive when someone mentions your drinking?

17. Do you become irritated when unexpected guests reduce your liquor supply?

18. Do you drink when under pressure or after an argument?

19. Do you try to cover up when you can't remember promises and feel ashamed when you misplace or lose things?

20. Do you drive even though you've been drinking, but feel certain you are in complete control of yourself?

Any woman who answers yes to more than half of these questions is probably alcoholic.

Treatment and Information Resources

Where to Write for Help in Finding Local Alcoholism Services

Alcoholics Anonymous World Services
PO Box 459
Grand Central Station
New York, New York 10017

Al-Anon Family Group Headquarters
P.O. Box 182
Madison Square Station
New York, New York 10010

Association of Halfway House Alcoholism Programs of North
America, Inc.
786 East 7th Street
St. Paul, Minnesota 55106

National Council on Alcoholism
12 West 21st Street
New York, New York 10010

The Other Victims of Alcoholism
P.O. Box 921 Radio City Station
New York, New York 10101

Women for Sobriety, Inc.
PO Box 618
Quakertown, Pennsylvania 18951

In Canada

Alcoholics Anonymous
272 Eglinton West
Toronto, Ontario

Alcoholics Anonymous
190 de Castelnau East
Montreal, Quebec

Most local areas have their own organizations dealing with the
problem; these are usually listed in the telephone book.

Notes

1. Superior But Not Equal

1. A. P. McKinlay, "The Roman Attitude Toward Women's Drinking," in *Drinking and Intoxication*, ed. R. G. McCarthy (New Haven: College and University Press, 1959).
2. S. B. Pomeroy, *Goddesses, Whores, Wives and Slaves—Women in Classical Antiquity* (New York: Schocken Books, 1975), p. 154.
3. J. Fraser, *The Female Alcoholic* (Toronto: Addiction Research Foundation, 1974), p. 3.
4. J. H. Hertz, ed., *Pentateuch and Haftorahs* (London: Soncino Press, 1970), p. 291.

2. Drinking Habits

1. A. P. McKinlay, "The Classical World," in *Drinking and Intoxication*, ed. R. G. McCarthy (New Haven: College and University Press, 1959).
2. From "Where the Souses Are," *Fortune*, March 1977.
3. F. L. Fitz-Gerald, "Voluntary Alcohol Consumption in Apes," in *Biology of Alcohol*, ed. D. Kissin and H. Begleiter, vol. 2 (New York: Plenum Publishing, 1972).
4. For further information on Native American Indians and alcohol, see J. Leland's *Firewater Myths* (New Brunswick: Rutgers Center of Alcohol Studies, 1976).
5. F. D. Harper, ed., *Alcohol Abuse and Black America* (Alexandria, Va: Douglass Publishers, 1974).

215

6. S. Nowell-Smith, ed., *Edwardian England 1901–1914* (London: Oxford University Press, 1964), p. 193.

7. From "High Court Bars Difference by Sex in Minimum Age for Buying Beer," *New York Times,* December 21, 1976.

3. EFFECTS ON BODY AND BRAIN

1. J. Horn, "Diet, Exercise and Alcohol: A Dangerous Combination," *Psychology Today,* January 1975, p. 26.

2. J. L. Arehart, "How Genes Control Drugs," *Science News* 99 (June 26, 1971): 438–39.

3. "The Advantages of Vitamin C," *New York Times,* July 3, 1977, p. E-6.

4. D. Goodwin, *Is Alcoholism Hereditary?* (New York: Oxford University Press, 1976), p. 8.

5. O. H. Rundell et al., "Alcohol and Sleep in Young Adults," *Psychopharmacologia* 26 (1972): 201–18.

6. M. Pines, "Speak, Memory: The Riddle of Recall and Forgetfulness," *Saturday Review,* August 9, 1975, p. 16.

7. R. C. Smith, E. S. Parker, and E. Noble, "Alcohol's Effect on Some Formal Aspects of Verbal Social Communication," *Archives of General Psychiatry* 32(1975): 1394–98.

8. B. M. Jones, "Verbal and Spatial Intelligence in Short and Long Term Alcoholics," *Journal of Nervous and Mental Disease* 153, no. 4 (1971): 292–97.

9. R. E. La Porte, et al., "Public Health Implications of Moderate Alcohol Consumption," *Journal of Public Health* 21 (1981): 198–223.

10. A. B. Lowenfils, "Alcoholism and the Risk of Cancer," *Medical Consequences of Alcoholism,* Annals of the New York Academy of Medicine, 252 (1975).

11. R. Athanasiou, P. Shaver, and C. Tavris, "Sex," *Psychology Today* 4 (1970): 37–52.

12. E. S. Gomberg, "Women and Alcoholism," in *Women in Therapy,* ed. V. Frank and V. Burtle (New York: Brunner/Mazel, 1974).

4. THE FIGHT AGAINST DEMON RUM

1. P. Smith, *Daughters of the Promised Land* (Boston: Little, Brown and Co., 1970), p. 118.

2. A. A. Gordon, *The Beautiful Life of Frances Willard* (Chicago: Woman's Temperance Publishing Assoc., 1898), p. 32.

3. M. Gurko, *The Ladies of Seneca Falls* (New York: Macmillan Publishing Co., 1974), p. 163.

5. WHO BECOMES ALCOHOLIC?

1. S. C. Wilsnack et al., "Drinking and Drinking Problems among Women in a U.S. National Survey," *Alcohol Health and Research World* 9, no. 2 (Winter 1984/85): 11.

2. Quoted in D. Cahalan, *Problem Drinkers* (San Francisco: Jossey-Bass, Inc., 1970), p. 5.

3. L. J. Beckman, "Women Alcoholics: A Review of Social and Psychological Studies," *Journal of Studies on Alcohol* 36, 1975, 797–825.

4. E. S. Gomberg, *Alcoholism and Women: State of Knowledge Today* (New York: National Council on Alcoholism, 1975).

5. M. A. Schuckit and E. R. Morrissey, "Alcoholism in Women: Some Clinical and Social Perspectives," in *Alcoholism Problems in Women and Children*, ed. M. Greenblatt and M. A. Schuckit (New York: Grune and Stratton, 1976), p. 11.

6. J. L. Arehart, "How Genes Control Drugs," *Science News* 99, June 26, 1971, 438–39.

7. R. Zucker, "Parental Influences Upon Drinking Patterns of Their Children," in *Alcoholism Problems in Women and Children*, ed. M. Greenblatt and M. A. Schuckit (New York: Grune and Stratton, 1976), pp. 47–48.

8. C. Wilsnack, "The Impact of Sex Roles on Women's Alcohol Use and Abuse," in *Alcoholism Problems in Women and Children*, ed. M. Greenblatt and M. A. Schuckit (New York: Grune and Stratton, 1976), pp. 47–48.

9. Ibid., p. 49.

10. H. Busch, E. Kormendy, and W. Feverlein, "Partners of Female Alcoholics," *British Journal of Addictions* 68 (1973): 179–84.

11. L. Fifield, quoted in *Alcohol Abuse Among Women: Special Problems and Unmet Needs*, U.S. Senate Hearing, September 29, 1976, p. 130.

6. FOR WOMEN ONLY

1. B. M. Jones and M. Jones, "Women and Alcohol: Intoxication, Metabolism and the Menstrual Cycle," in *Alcoholism Problems in Women and Children*, ed. M. Greenblatt and M. A. Schuckit (New York: Grune and Stratton, 1976).

2. B. M. Jones and M. Jones, "Interaction of Alcohol, Oral Contraceptives and the Menstrual Cycle with Stimulus-Response Compatibility," in *Currents in Alcoholism*, ed. F. A. Seixas, vol. 2 (New York: Grune and Stratton, 1977).

3. M. K. Jones and B. M. Jones, "Alcohol Metabolism in Women on Oral Contraceptives," Second Oklahoma Symposium on Drinking Behavior and Alcoholism, Oklahoma City, December 9, 1976.

4. A. W. Marshall et al., "Ethanol Elimination in Males and Females: Relationship to Menstrual Cycle and Body Composition," *Hepatology* 3, no. 5 (1983): 701–06.

5. S. Wilsnack, "Sex Role Identity in Female Alcoholism," *Journal of Abnormal Psychology* 82 (1973): 253–61.

6. M. Valimaki and R. Ylikahri, "Effect of Alcohol on Male and Female Sexual Function," *Alcohol and Alcoholism* 18, no. 4 (1983): 313–20.

7. H. D. Archibald, *Toward Saturation in Search of Control* (Toronto: Addiction Research Foundation, 1975), p. 10.

7. FOR MEDICINAL PURPOSES ONLY

1. From "A Vintage Medicine," *New York Times*, June 12, 1977, p. 21.

2. D. D. Reeves, "Come All for the Cure-All," *Harvard Library Bulletin* 15, no. 3 (July 1967).

3. For more about Lydia Pinkham, see J. Burton's biography, *Lydia Pinkham Is Her Name* (New York: Farrar, Strauss and Co., 1949).

4. J. H. Young, *The Toadstool Millionaires* (Princeton: Princeton University Press, 1961), p. 104.

5. National Institute on Drug Abuse Conference, *Drugs, Alcohol and*

Women (Washington D.C.: National Research and Communications Association, Inc., 1975), p. 145.

6. E. P. Noble quoted in *The Alcoholism Report* 5, no. 12 (April 8, 1977): 3.

8. ALCOHOL AND THE FAMILY

1. *The Whole College Catalog About Drinking* (Washington D.C.: U.S. Department of Health, Education and Welfare, 1976), p. 2.

2. A. Paredes, "Marital-Sexual Factors in Alcoholism," *Medical Aspects of Human Sexuality* (April 1973): 98–115.

3. *Alcohol Health and Research World* (National Institute on Alcohol Abuse and Alcoholism, Washington, D.C., 9, no. 1 (Fall 1984): 34.

4. M. A. Schuckit and E. Morrisey, "Alcoholism in Women: Some Clinical and Social Perspectives with an Emphasis on Possible Subtypes" in *Alcoholism Problems in Women and Children*, ed. M. Greenblatt and M. A. Schuckit (New York: Grune and Stratton, 1976): 17.

5. J. Albon, "Al-Anon Family Groups," *American Journal of Psychotherapy* 28, no. 1 (January 1974): 30–45.

6. M. Bohman et al., "Maternal Inheritance of Alcohol Abuse: Cross Fostering Analysis of Adopted Women," *Archives of General Psychiatry* 38 (1981): 965–69.

7. R. Zucker, "Parental Influences Upon Drinking Patterns of Their Children," in *Alcoholism Problems in Women and Children*, ed. M. Greenblatt and M. A. Schuckit (New York: Grune and Stratton, 1976).

9. ALCOHOL AND PREGNANCY

1. J. W. Hanson, K. L. Jones, and D. W. Smith, "Fetal Alcohol Syndrome, Experience with 41 Patients," *Journal of the American Medical Association* 235 (1976): 1458–60.

2. A. B. Mukherjee et al., "Maternal Ethanol Exposure Induces Transient Impairment of Umbilical Circulation and Fetal Hypoxia in Monkeys," *Science* 218, no. 12 (November 1982): 700–02.

3. J. L. Mills et al., "Maternal Alcohol Consumption and Birth Weight: How Much Drinking During Pregnancy Is Too Much?" *Journal of the American Medical Association* 252, no. 14 (October 12, 1984): 1875–79.

4. A. P. Streissguth, "Female Alcoholism: Impacts on Women and Children," in *Currents in Alcoholism*, ed. M. Galanter, vol. 7 (Orlando, Fla.: Grune and Stratton, 1980).

5. K. L. Jones et al., "Outcome of Offspring in Alcoholic Women," *Lancet* 1 (1974): 1076–78.

6. G. Gordon et al., "Effect of Alcohol (Ethanol) Administration on Sex-Hormone Metabolism in Normal Men," *New England Journal of Medicine* 295, no. 5 (1976): 796–97.

10. TREATMENT OF ALCOHOLISM

1. R. J. Gibbins et al., ed., *Research Advances in Alcohol and Drug Problems*, vol. 2 (New York: John Wiley and Sons, 1975), p. 280.

2. J. Curlee, "Sex Differences in Patient Attitudes Toward Alcoholism Treatment," *Quarterly Journal of Studies on Alcohol* 32 (1971): 643–50.

3. N. Grey, "Survey: Women's Problems," *Drug Survival News*, June 1977, p. 7.

4. D. A. Thomas, "A Study of Selective Factors of Successfully and Non-Successfully Treated Women Alcoholics," *Dissertation Abstracts* 32 (1971): 1862–63.

5. E. J. Larkin, *The Treatment of Alcoholism: Theory, Practice and Evaluation* (Ontario: Addiction Research Foundation, 1974), p. 33.

6. H. F. Krimmel and D. B. Falkey, "Short-Term Treatment of Alcoholics," *Social Work* 7, no. 1 (1962): 102–07.

7. A. I. Alterman et al., "Consequences of Social Modification of Drinking Behavior," *Journal of Studies on Alcohol* 38, no. 5 (1977): 1032.

Bibliography

Ablon, J. "Al-Anon Family Groups." *American Journal of Psychotherapy* 27 (January 1974): 30–45.

Alcohol Abuse Among Women: Special Problems and Unmet Needs. U.S. Senate Hearing: September 29, 1976.

The Alcohol, Drug Abuse, and Mental Health National Data Book, U.S. Department of Health, Education and Welfare, January 1980 Publication Number (ADM) 80–938.

Alcohol and Health. Washington, D.C.: U.S. Department of Health, Education and Welfare, December 1971.

Alcohol and Health. Washington, D.C.: U.S. Department of Health, Education and Welfare, 1978.

Alcohol and Health: New Knowledge. Washington, D.C.: U.S. Department of Health, Education and Welfare, June 1974.

Alcohol Health and Research World. Washington, D.C.: National Institute on Alcohol Abuse and Alcoholism, 9, no. 1 (Fall 1984): 37.

"Alcohol Indicted as Strong Teratogen." *Medical World News* (September 19, 1977): 15.

Alexander, C. N., et al. "Peer Influences on Adolescent Drinking." *Quarterly Journal of Studies on Alcohol* 28 (1967).

Alibrandi, T., et al. "Drinking Patterns and Problem Drinking Among Youth in Orange County." Presented at The National Council on Alcoholism Forum, 29 April–4 May 1977.

Allen, F. L. *Only Yesterday.* New York: Harper and Bros., 1931.

Alterman, A. I., et al. "Consequences of Social Modification of Drinking Behavior." *Journal of Studies on Alcohol* 38 (1977): 1032.

Annis, H., and Liban, C. "Alcoholism in Women: Treatment Modalities and Outcomes." *Alcohol and Drug Problems in Women* 5. Edited by O. H. Kalant. New York: Plenum Publishing, 1980, 385–422.

Archibald, H. D. *Toward Saturation—In Search of Control.* Toronto: Addiction Research Foundation, 1975.

Arehart, Joan Lynn. "How Genes Control Drugs." *Science News* 99, June 26, 1971, 438–39.

Argeriou, M., et al. "Women Arrested for Drunken Driving in Boston, Social Characteristics and Circumstances of Arrest." *Journal of Studies on Alcohol* 37 (May 1976): 648.

Armor, D. J., et al. *Alcoholism and Treatment.* Santa Monica, Cal.: Rand Corporation, June 1976.

Arnaldus of Villanova. *The Earliest Printed Book on Wine.* Translated by Henry E. Sigerist, M.D. New York: Schuman's, 1953.

Athanasiou, P. et al. "Sex." *Psychology Today* 4 (1970): 37–52.

Bacon, S. D. "Classic Temperance Movement of the U.S.A.: Impact Today on Attitudes, Action and Research." *British Journal of Addictions* 62 (1967): 5–18.

Bailey, M. B., et al. "Normal Drinking in Persons Reporting Previous Problem Drinking." *Quarterly Journal of Studies on Alcohol* 28 (1967): 305–15.

Bailey, Ronald H. *The Role of the Brain.* New York: Time-Life Books, 1975.

Baillargeon, J., et al. "Alcoholism Treatment Programming: Historical Trends and Modern Approaches." *Alcoholism: Clinical and Experimental Research* 1 (October 1977): 311–18.

Batterberry, Michael. *On the Town in New York.* New York: Charles Scribner's Sons, 1973.

Beckman, L. J. "Alcoholism Problems and Women: An Overview." *Alcoholism Problems in Women and Children.* Edited by M. Greenblatt and M. A. Schuckit, New York: Grune and Stratton, 1976.

Benion, L. J. "Alcohol Metabolism in American Indians and Whites." *New England Journal of Medicine* 249 (1976): 24.

Bissell, L. "The Treatment of Alcoholism: What Do We Do About Long-Term Sedatives?" *Annals of the New York Academy of Sciences* 252 (1975): 396–99.

———, et al. "The Smithers Center Treating the Urban Alcoholic." *P and S Quarterly* 21 (Spring 1974): 13–16.

Blane, H. T. *The Personality of the Alcoholic: Guises of Dependency.* New York: Harper & Row, 1968.

Blume, S. D. "Iatrogenic Alcoholism." *Quarterly Journal of Studies on Alcohol* 34 (December 1973): 1348–52.

Bohman, M., et al. "Maternal Inheritance of Alcohol Abuse: Cross Fostering Analysis of Adopted Women." *Archives of General Psychiatry* 38: 965–69.

Bowen, M. "Alcoholism As Viewed Through Family Systems Theory and Family Psychotherapy." *The Person With Alcoholism.* Edited by F. A. Seixas, R. Cadoret, and S. Eggleston. New York: *Annals of the New York Academy of Sciences* 223 (1974): 115–22.

Brewin, T. B. "The Incidence of Alcohol Intolerance in Women with Tumors of the Uterus, Ovary, or Breast." *Proceedings of the Royal Society of Medicine* 60 (December 1967): 1308–09.

Burgess, Louise Bailey. *Alcohol and Your Health.* Los Angeles: Charles Publishing, 1973.

Burton, Jean. *Lydia Pinkham Is Her Name.* New York: Farrar, Straus, 1949.

Busch, H., et al. "Partners of Female Alcoholics." *British Journal of Addictions* 68)1973): 179–84.

Cahalan, D. *Problem Drinkers.* San Francisco: Jossey-Bass, Inc., 1970.

————, et al. *American Drinking Practices: A National Study of Drinking Behavior and Attitudes.* New Haven: College and University Press Services, 1969.

Chafe, William. *The American Woman: Her Changing Social Roles.* New York: Oxford University Press, 1974.

Chafetz, M. E. *Liquor, the Servant of Man.* Boston: Little, Brown and Co., 1965.

————. *Why Drinking Can Be Good For You.* New York: Stein and Day, 1976.

Chandler, B. C., et al. "Altered Hemispheric Functioning Under Alcohol." *Journal of Studies on Alcohol* 38 (March): 381–91.

Chidsey, Donald Barr. *On and Off the Wagon.* New York: Cowles Book Co., 1969 (2): 159, 1977.

Clark, W. B., and Midanik, L. "Alcohol Use and Alcohol Problems Among U. S. Adults: Results of the 1979 National Survey." *Alcohol and Health Monograph* no. 1. Washington, D.C.: National Institute on Alcohol Abuse and Alcoholism, 1982.

Clarren, S. K., et al. "Brain Malformations in Human Offspring Exposed to Alcohol in Utero." *Alcoholism: Clinical and Experimental Research,* 1978.

————. "The Fetal Alcohol Syndrome." *New England Journal of Medicine,* 298: 1063.

Cork, Margaret. *The Forgotten Children.* Toronto: Addiction Research Foundation, 1969.

Corrigan, E. M. *Alcoholic Women in Treatment.* New York: Oxford University Press, 1980.

————. "Women and Problem Drinking: Notes on Beliefs and Facts." *Addictive Diseases* 1 (1974): 215.

Costello, R. M., et al. "Alcoholism Treatment Programming: Historical Trends and Modern Approaches." *Alcoholism: Clinical and Experimental Research* 1, no. 4, October 1977.

Council of Scientific Affairs. "Fetal Effects of Maternal Alcohol Use." *Journal of the American Medical Association* 245, no. 18 (May 13, 1983): 2517–21.

Critical Review of the Fetal Alcohol Syndrome. Washington, D.C.: National Institute on Alcohol Abuse and Alcoholism, 1977.

Curlee, Jean. "A Comparison of Male and Female Patients at an Alcoholism Treatment Center." *Journal of Psychology* 74 (1970): 239–47.

————. "Alcoholism and the 'Empty Nest.' " Bulletin 33 of the Menninger Clinic (1969): 165–71.

————. "Sex Differences in Patient Attitudes Toward Alcoholism Treatment." *Quarterly Journal of Studies on Alcohol* 32: 643–50.

Day, N. "Estimates of the Role of Alcohol in Mortality." *Drinking and Drug Practices Surveyor,* no. 11 (1976): 18–23.

Doherty, J. "Disulfiram (Antabuse): Chemical Commitment to Abstinence." *Alcohol Health and Research World* (Spring 1976): 2–7.

"Drinking Troubles More Families." *The New York Times,* February 13, 1977.

Drugs, Alcohol and Women. National Institute on Drug Abuse Conference. Washington, D.C.: National Research and Communications Association, 1975.

Drugs and American High School Students 1975–1983. Rockville, Md.: National Institute on Drug Abuse, 1984.

DuPont, R. L. "Drugs, Alcohol and Women." *Vital Speeches of the Day* (1975): 140–43.

Edwards, G., et al. "Alcoholism: A Controlled Trial of 'Treatment' and 'Advice.' " *Journal of Studies on Alcohol* 38 (1977): 1004–22.

Edwards, H. *Dionysius.* New York: Macmillan, 1965.

Eisenstein, V. W., ed. *Neurotic Interaction in Marriage.* New York: Basic Books, 1956.

Engs, R. C. "Drinking Patterns and Drinking Problems of College Students." *Journal of Studies on Alcohol* 38 (1977): 2144–56.

Epstein, P. S., et al. "Alcoholism and Cerebral Atrophy." *Alcoholism: Clinical and Experimental Research* 1 (January 1977): 61–65.

Fifield, L. Quoted in *Alcohol Abuse Among Women: Special Problems and Unmet Needs.* U.S. Senate Hearing, September 29, 1976.

Fillmore, K. M. "Drinking and Problem Drinking in Early Adulthood and Middle Age." *Quarterly Journal of Studies on Alcohol* 35 (1974): 819–40.

Fisher, Arthur. "Sober—Yet Drinking Too Much." *New York Times Magazine,* May 18, 1975.

Fitzgerald, B. J., et al. "Four-Year Follow Up Study of Alcoholics Treated at a Rural State Hospital." *Quarterly Journal of Studies on Alcohol* 32 (1971): 636.

Fort, Joel, M.D. *Alcohol: Our Biggest Drug Problem.* New York: McGraw-Hill, 1973.

Fortune, "Where The Souses Are." (March, 1977).

Fourth Special Report to the U.S. Congress on Alcohol and Health. Washington, D.C.: U.S. Department of Health and Human Services, January 1981.

Fox, Ruth. "The Alcoholic Spouse." *Neurotic Interaction in Marriage.* Edited By V. W. Eisenstein. New York: Basic Books, 1956.

———, et al. *Alcoholism: Its Scope, Cause and Treatment.* New York: Random House, 1955.

Fox, V., et al. "Evaluation of a Chemo-Therapeutic Program for the Rehabilitation of Alcoholics: Observations Over a Two Year Period." *Quarterly Journal of Studies on Alcohol* 20 (1959): 767–80.

Fraser, Judy. *The Female Alcoholic.* Toronto: Addiction Research Foundation, 1976.

Fraser, W. "The Alcoholic Woman: Attitudes and Perspectives." *Women: Their Use of Alcohol and Other Legal Drugs.* Edited by Anne MacLennan. Toronto: Addiction Research Foundation, 1976.

Fuchs, A. R. "The Inhibitory Effect of Ethanol on the Release of Oxytocin During Parturition in the Rabbit." *Journal of Endocrinology* 35 (1966): 125–34.

Fuchs, F., et al. "Effect of Alcohol in Threatened Premature Labor." *American Journal of Obstetrics and Gynecology* 99 (1967): 627–37.

Furnas, J. C. *The Life and Times of the Late Demon Rum.* New York: G. P. Putnam's Sons, 1965.

Garrett, G. R. "Women on Skid Row." *Quarterly Journal of Studies on Alcohol* 34 (1973): 1228–43.

Gerard, D. L. "Intoxication and Addiction." *Quarterly Journal of Studies on Alcohol* 16 (1955): 681–89.

Gibbins, R. J., et al., eds. *Research Advances in Alcohol and Drug Problems.* Vol. 2. New York: John Wiley and Sons, 1975.

Glover, J. H. "Electrical Aversion Therapy with Alcoholics: A Comparative Follow Up Study." *British Journal of Psychiatry* 130 (1977): 279–86.

Gomberg, E. S. *Alcoholism and Women: State of Knowledge Today.* New York: National Council on Alcoholism, 1975.

———. "Women and Alcoholism." *Women in Therapy.* Edited by V. Franks and V. Burtle. New York: Brunner/Mazel, 1974.

———. "Women with Alcohol Problems." *Alcoholism: Development, Consequences and Interventions.* Edited by N. J. Estes and M. E. Heinemann. St. Louis: C. V. Mosby, 1977.

Goodwin, D. W. *Is Alcoholism Hereditary?* New York: Oxford University Press, 1976.

———, et al. "Alcoholism and Depression in Adopted-Out Daughters of Alcoholics." *Archives of General Psychiatry* 34 (July 1977): 751–55.

Gordon, A. A. *The Beautiful Life of Frances Willard.* Chicago: Woman's Temperance Publishing Assoc., 1898.

Gordon, G., et al. "Effect of Alcohol (Ethanol) Administration on Sex-Hormone Metabolism in Normal Men." *New England Journal of Medicine* 295 (1976): 796–97.

Grey, Nancy. "Survey: Women's Problems." *Drug Survival News* (June 1977): 7.

Gurko, M. *The Ladies of Seneca Falls.* New York: Macmillan, 1974.

Hanson, J. W. "Fetal Alcohol Syndrome, Experience With 41 Patients." *Journal of the American Medical Association* 235 (1976): 1458–60.

"Happy Talk." *Newsweek,* August 26, 1974, p. 89.

Harford, T. C. "Contextual Drinking Patterns Among Men and Women." Durham, N. C.: Research Triangle Institute, 1974.

Harper, F. D., ed. *Alcohol Abuse and Black America.* Alexandria, Va.: Douglass Publishers, 1974.

Hatcher, B. S., et al. "Cognitive Deficits in Alcoholic Women." *Alcoholism: Clinical and Experimental Research* 1 (October 1977).

Herodotus, "Persian Wars, Book II." *The Greek Historians* 1. Edited by F. R. B. Godolphin. New York: Random House, 1942, p. 106.

Hertz, J. H., ed. *Pentateuch and Haftorahs.* London: Soncino Press, 1970.

"Hic! Go Easy, Ladies." *London Daily Mirror,* June 10, 1977.

Hindman, Margaret. "Family Therapy in Alcoholism." *Alcohol Health and Research World* 1 (Fall 1976).

Homiller, Jonica D. *Women and Alcohol: A Guide For State and Local Decision Makers.* Washington, D.C.: American Drug Problems Association, 1977.

Horn, J. "Diet, Exercise and Alcohol: A Dangerous Combination." *Psychology Today* (January 1975): 26.

Horton, D. "Primitive Societies." *Drinking and Intoxication.* Edited by R. G. McCarthy. New Haven: College and University Press, 1959.

James, J. E. "Symptoms of Alcoholism in Women: A Preliminary Survey of A.A. Members." *Journal of Studies on Alcohol* 36 (1975).

Jellinek, E. M. *The Disease Concept of Alcoholism.* New Haven: College and University Press, 1960.

Johnson, Vernon. *I'll Quit Tomorrow.* New York: Harper & Row, 1973.

Jones, B. M. "Alcohol and Women: Intoxication Levels and Memory Impairment as Related to the Menstrual Cycle." *Alcohol Technical Reports* 4 (January 1975): 4–9.

———. "Circadian Variation in the Effects of Alcohol on Cognitive Performance." *Quarterly Journal of Studies on Alcohol* 35 (December 1974): 1212–19.

———. "Cognitive Performance of Introverts and Extroverts Following Acute Alcohol Ingestion." *British Journal of Psychology* 65 (1974): 35–42.

———. "Verbal and Spatial Intelligence in Short and Long Term Alcoholics." *Journal of Nervous and Mental Disease* 1953 (1971): 292–97.

———, et al. "Alcohol and Consciousness: Getting High: Coming Down." *Psychology Today* (January 1975): 53–58.

———, et al. "Interaction of Alcohol, Oral Contraceptives and the Menstrual Cycle With Stimulus-Response Compatability." *Currents in Alcoholism* II. Edited by F. A. Seixas. New York: Grune and Stratton, 1977.

———, et al. "Women and Alcohol: Intoxication, Metabolism and the Menstrual Cycle." *Alcoholism Problems in Women and Children.* Edited by M. Greenblatt and M. A. Schuckit. New York: Grune and Stratton, 1976.

Jones, K. L., et al. "Outcome of Offspring in Alcoholic Women." *Lancet* 1 (1974): 1076–78.

———, et al. "Pattern of Malformation in Offspring of Chronic Alcoholic Mothers." *Lancet* 1 (1973): 1267–71.

Jones, M. C. "Personality Antecedants and Correlates of Drinking Patterns in Women." *Journal of Consulting and Clinical Psychology* 36 (1971): 61–69.

Jones, M. K., and Jones, B. M. "Alcohol Metabolism in Women on Oral Contraceptives." Second Oklahoma Symposium on Drinking Behavior and Alcoholism. Oklahoma City, December 9, 1976.

Jones, R. W., et al. "Treatment of Alcoholism by Physicians in Private Practice." *Quarterly Journal of Studies on Alcohol* 32 (1971): 643–50.

Jung, John. "Drinking Motives and Behavior." *Journal of Studies on Alcohol* 38 (1977): 944–52.

Kanowitz, L. *Women and the Law.* Albuquerque: University of New Mexico Press, 1969.

Karpman, B. *The Hangover.* Springfield, Ill.: Charles C. Thomas, 1957.

Kent, Patricia. *An American Woman and Alcohol.* New York: Holt, Rinehart and Winston, 1967.

Kiev, Ari, M.D., ed. *Somatic Manifestations of Depressive Disorders.* Princeton: Excerpta Medica, 1974.

Kissin, D., and Begleiter, H. *Biology of Alcoholism.* Vol. 2. New York: Plenum Publishing, 1972.

Kitson, T. M. "The Disulfiram-Ethanol Reaction: A Review." *Journal of Studies on Alcohol* 38 (1977): 96–113.

Klatsky, A. L., et al. "Alcohol Consumption and Blood Pressure." *New England Journal of Medicine* 296 (May 26, 1977): 1194–1200.

Krimmel, H. F., et al. "Short Term Treatment of Alcoholics." *Social Work* 7 (1962): 102–07.

La Porte, R. E., et al. "Public Health Implications of Moderate Alcohol Consumption." *Journal of Public Health* 21 (1981): 198–223.

Larkin, E. J. *The Treatment of Alcoholism: Theory, Practice and Evaluation.* Toronto: Addiction Research Foundation, 1974.

Leake, D. Chauncy, et al. *Alcoholic Beverages in Clinical Medicine.* Chicago: Year Book Medical Publishers, 1966.

Leland, Joy, *Firewater Myths.* New Brunswick: Rutgers Center of Alcohol Studies, 1976.

LeMasters, E. E. *Blue-Collar Aristocrats.* Madison: University of Wisconsin Press, 1975.

Lemoine, P., et al. "Les Enfants de Parents Alcoöliques: Anomalies Observées à Propos de 127 cas [Children of Alcoholic Parents: Anomalies Observed in 127 cases]. *Ouest Medicine* 25 (1968): 476–82.

Lender, M. L., et al. "Temperance Tales." *Journal of Studies on Alcohol* 38 (1977): 1347–70.

Lerner, Gerda. "The Lady and the Mill Girl." *Women and Womanhood in America.* Compiled by R. W. Hogeland. Lexington, Mass.: D. C. Heath, 1973.

Lester, B. K., et al. "Chronic Alcoholism, Alcohol and Sleep." *Alcohol Intoxication and Withdrawal: Experimental Studies: Advances in Experimental Medicine* 5. Edited by M. Gross. New York: Plenum Publishing, 1973.

Lieber, C. "The Metabolism of Alcohol." *Scientific American,* March 1976, pp. 25–83.

Lisansky, E. T. "Alcoholism: A Symposium." *Georgetown Medical Bulletin* 27 (August 1973): 7–23.

Little, R., et al. "Drinking During Pregnancy." *Journal of Studies on Alcohol* 37 (1976): 375–79.

Loehlin, J. S. "Nature and Nurture in Alcoholism." *Annals of the New York Academy of Sciences* 197 (1972): 117–20.

Lowenfils, A. B. "Alcoholism and the Risk of Cancer." *Medical Consequences of Alcoholism.* Annals of the New York Academy of Medicine, 252 (1975).

Lowenfish, Sonja K. *The Woman Alcoholic—Her Clinical and Social Emergence.* Quakertown, Pa: Women for Sobriety, 1976.

Lucia, Salvatore P., M.D. *A History of Wine As Therapy.* Philadelphia: J. B. Lippincott, 1963.

Lynd, R. S., et al. *Middletown in Transition.* New York: Harcourt, Brace and World, 1937.

Lynes, Russell. *Snobs.* New York: Harper and Bros., 1950.

MacAndrew, C., et al. *Drunken Comportment.* Chicago: Aldine Publishing Co., 1969.

McClelland, David, et al. "The Drinking Man." *Social Scientists.* New York: The Free Press, 1972.

McIlroy, A. L. "The Influence of Alcohol and Alcoholism on Ante-natal and Infant Life." *British Journal of Inebriety* 21 (1923): 39–42.

McKinlay, A. P. "Bacchus as Health Giver." *Quarterly Journal of Studies on Alcohol* 11 (1950): 230–46.

———. "The Classical World." *Drinking and Intoxication.* Edited by R. G. McCarthy. New Haven: College and University Press, 1959.

———. "The Roman Attitude Toward Women's Drinking." *Drinking and Intoxication.*

Mahoney, Barbara. *A Sensitive, Passionate Man.* New York: David McKay, Inc., 1974.

Malcolm, John. *The History of Persia.* Vol. 1. London: 1815.

Mann, M. *New Primer on Alcoholism.* New York: Holt, Rinehart and Winston, 1958.

Marshall, A. W., et al. "Ethanol Elimination in Males and Females: Relationship to Menstrual Cycle and Body Composition." *Hepatology* 3, no. 5 (1983): 701–06.

Medhus, A. "Mortality Among Female Alcoholics." *Scandinavian Journal of Social Medicine* 3 (1975): 535–47.

Merryman, Richard. *Broken Promises, Mended Dreams.* Boston: Little, Brown, and Co., 1984.

Miller, W. R., et al. "Abstinence and Controlled Drinking in the Treatment of Problem Drinkers." *Journal of Studies on Alcohol* 38 (1977): 986–1003.

Mishara, B. L., et al. "Alcohol's Effects in Old Age: An Experimental Investigation." *Social Science and Medicine* 9 (1975): 535–47.

Mills, James L., et al. "Maternal Alcohol Consumption and Birth Weight: How Much Drinking During Pregnancy Is Too Much?" *Journal of the American Medical Association* 252, no. 14 (October 12, 1984): 1875–79.

Morrissey, E. R., and Schuckit, M. A. "Stressful Life Events and Alcoholism in Women Seen in a Detoxification Center." Manuscript.

Mukherjee, A. B., et al. "Maternal Ethanol Exposure Induces Transient Impairment of Umbilical Circulation and Fetal Hypoxia in Monkeys." *Science* 218 (November 12, 1982): 700–02.

Myers, R. D., et al. "Alcohol Drinking: Abnormal Intake Caused by Tetrahydropapaveroline in the Brain." *Science* 196 (April 29, 1977): 554–55.

Nellis, M., et al. "Final Report on Drugs, Alcohol and Women's Health." Mimeographed report. Washington, D.C.: National Research Communications Association, Inc., 1978.

New York Times, "A Vintage Medicine," June 12, 1977.

Noble, E. P., et al. "Alcohol Induced Changes in Brain Protein Synthesis." Abstracted in *Alcoholism: Clinical and Experimental Research* 1, no. 2, April 1977.

——. Quoted in *The Alcoholism Report* 5, no. 12 (April 18, 1977): 3.

Norris, John. Quoted in Weisman, Maxwell N., M.D., "Book Reviews." *Alcohol and Health Research World.* (Spring 1976): 27.

Nowell-Smith, Simon, ed. *Edwardian England 1901–1914.* London: Oxford University Press, 1964.

O'Brien, R., and Chafetz, M. *The Encyclopedia of Alcoholism.* New York: Facts on File Publications, 1982.

O'Donnell, J. "They're Drinking More Than Ever." *Collier's Weekly* 73 (June 21, 1924): 9.

Ouellette, E. M., et al. "Adverse Effects on Offspring of Maternal Alcohol Abuse During Pregnancy." *New England Journal of Medicine* 297 (1977): 528–30.

Pandina, R., ed. "Coping with Adolescent Substance Abuse." Rutgers University.

Paredes, A. "Future Plans and Goals in Research: The Oklahoma Center of Alcohol and Drug-Related Studies." *Annals of the New York Academy of Sciences* 273 (May 28, 1976): 103–09.

——. "Marital-Sexual Factors in Alcoholism." *Medical Aspects of Human Sexuality* (April 1973): 98–115.

——, et al. "Loss of Control in Alcoholism: An Investigation of the Hypothesis, With Experimental Findings." *Quarterly Journal of Studies on Alcohol* 34 (1973): 1146–61.

Parker, E., et al. "Alcohol Consumption and Cognitive Functioning in Social Drinking." *Quarterly Journal of Studies on Alcohol* 38 (1977) 1224–32.

Partanen, J. "On the Relevance of Twin Studies." *Annals of the New York Academy of Sciences* 197 (1972): 117–20.

Pearl, Raymond. *Alcohol and Longevity.* New York: Alfred A. Knopf, 1926.

Pfautz, W. H. "The Image of Alcohol in Popular Fiction: 1900–1904 and 1946–1950." *Quarterly Journal of Studies in Alcohol* 23 (1962): 131–46.

Pines, Maya. "Speak, Memory: The Riddle of Recall and Forgetfulness." *Saturday Review,* August 9, 1975, p. 16.

Pittman, David J., and Snyder, Charles R., eds. *Society, Culture and Drinking Patterns*. Carbondale and Edwardsville: Southern Illinois University Press, 1962.

Pomeroy, S. B. *Goddesses, Whores, Wives and Slaves—Women in Classical Antiquity*. New York: Schocken Books, 1975.

"Preliminary Summary: Surveillance of Student Drug Use." San Mateo Department of Public Health and Welfare, 1973.

Putnam, E. J. *The Lady*. Chicago: University of Chicago Press, 1970.

Rachal, J. V., et al. "A National Study of Adolescent Drinking Behavior, Attitudes and Correlates." Durham, N.C.: Research Triangle Institute, 1975.

Randall, C. L., et al. "Ethanol-induced Malformations in Mice." *Alcoholism: Clinical and Experimental Research* 1 (1977): 219–23.

Rebeta-Burditt, Joyce. *The Cracker Factory*. New York: Macmillan, 1977.

Reeves, D. D. "Come All For The Cure All." *Harvard Library Bulletin* 15 (July 1967).

Reeves, N. *Womankind Beyond the Stereotypes*. Chicago: Aldine-Atherton, 1971.

"Report on the International Council of Women." Washington, D.C.: The National Woman Suffrage Assoc. March 25–April 1, 1888.

Roizen, R. "Comment on the Rand Report." *Journal of Studies on Alcohol* 38 (January 1977): 170–78.

Room, R. "Drinking Patterns in Large U.S. Cities: A Comparison of San Francisco and National Samples." *Quarterly Journal of Studies on Alcohol Supplement No. 6* (1972): 1–27.

Rosin, A. J., et al. "Alcohol Excess in the Elderly." *Quarterly Journal of Studies on Alcohol* 32 (1971): 52–59.

Roueché, Berton. "Cultural Factors and Drinking Patterns." *Annals of the American Academy of Science* 133 (1966): 787–882.

Rubington, Earl. "The Hidden Alcoholic." *Quarterly Journal of Studies on Alcohol* 33 (1972): 667–81.

Rundell, O. H., et al. "Alcohol and Sleep in Young Adults." *Psychopharmacologia* 26 (1972): 201–18.

Sadoun, R., et al. *Drinking in French Culture*. New Brunswick, N.J.: Rutgers Center of Alcohol Studies, 1965.

Saghir, M. T., et al. "Homosexuality IV, Psychiatric Disorders and Disability in the Female Alcoholic." *American Journal of Psychiatry* 127 (1970): 147–54.

Sandmaier, Marian. *Alcohol Abuse and Women: A Guide to Getting Help*. Rockville, Md.: National Institute on Alcohol Abuse and Alcoholism, 1976.

———. *The Invisible Alcoholics. Women and Alcohol Abuse in America*. New York: McGraw-Hill, 1980.

Saville, P. D. "Alcoholism-Related Skeletal Disorders." *Annals of the New York Academy of Sciences* 252 (1975).

———. "The Alcoholic Woman: A Literature Review." *Psychiatric Medicine* 3 (1972): 37–43.

Schuckit, M. A. "A Short Term Follow Up of Women Alcoholics." *Diseases of the Nervous System* 33 (October 1972): 672–78.

———, et al. "Alcoholism in Women: Some Clinical and Social Perspectives." *Alcoholism Problems in Women and Children*. New York: Grune and Stratton, 1976.

————, et al. "Alcoholism: Two Types of Alcoholism in Women." *Archives of Environmental Health* 18 (March 1969): 301–06.

Seixas, F. A. "Alcohol and Its Drug Interactions." *Annals of Internal Medicine* 83 (July 1975): 86–92.

————. "Treating Alcoholics: A Practical Program for Family Physicians." *Medical Times* 99 (July 1971): 45–58.

Seixas, J., and Youcha, G. *Children of Alcoholism: A Survivor's Manual.* New York: Crown Publishers, Inc., 1985.

Senseman, L. I. "The Housewife's Secret Illness: How to Recognize the Female Alcoholic." *Rhode Island Medical Journal* 49 (1966): 40–42.

Sexton, P. C. "Speaking For the Working Class Wife." *Harper's*, October 1962.

Shaw, S., et al. "Plasma Alpha Amino-n-Butyric Acid to Leucine Ratio: An Empirical Biochemical Marker of Alcoholism." *Science* 18 (December 3, 1976): 1057–58.

Smith, P. *Daughters of the Promised Land.* Boston: Little, Brown, and Co., 1970.

Smith, R. C., et al. "Alcohol's Effects on Some Formal Aspects of Verbal Social Communication." *Archives of General Psychiatry* 32 (1975), 1394–98.

Steiner, Claude, M.D. *Games Alcoholics Play.* New York: Grove Press, 1971.

Stevens, Elizabeth. *Babbitts and Bohemians.* New York: Macmillan, 1967.

Streissguth, A. P. "Female Alcoholism: Impacts on Women and Children." *Currents in Alcoholism* 7. Edited by M. Galanter. New York: Grune and Stratton, in press.

Talbott, G. D. "Primary Alcoholic Heart Disease." *Annals of the New York Academy of Sciences* 252 (1975): 237–39.

Tamerin, J. S., et al. "The Upper-Class Alcoholic; A Syndrome in Itself?" *Psychosomatics* 12 (1971): 200–04.

Taylor, R. L. *Vessel of Wrath—Carry Nation.* New York: Signet, 1966.

Thomas, D. A. "A Study of Selective Factors of Successfully and Non-Successfully Treated Alcoholics." *Dissertation Abstracts* 32 (1971): 1862–63.

Tracey, D. A., et al. "Behavioral Analysis of Chronic Alcoholism in Four Women." *Journal of Consulting and Clinical Psychology* 44 (1976): 832–42.

U.S. Bureau of the Census, Statistical Abstract of the U.S. (105th edition), Washington, D.C., 1984.

Valimaki, M., and Ylikahri, R. "Effect of Alcohol on Male and Female Sexual Function." *Alcohol and Alcoholism* 18, no. 4 (1983): 313–20.

Wallgren, H., et al. *Actions of Alcohol.* New York: Elsevier Publishing Co., 1970.

Wanberg, K. W., et al. "Alcohol Use Inventory." *Journal of Studies on Alcohol* 38 (March 1977): 512–43.

————, et al. "Alcoholism Symptom Patterns of Men and Women: A Comparative Study." *Quarterly Journal of Studies on Alcohol* 31 (1970) 40–61.

Warner, R. H., et al. "The Effect of Drinking on Offspring: A Historical Survey of American and British Literature." *Journal of Studies on Alcohol* 36 (1975): 1395–1420.

Washburne, Chandler. *Primitive Drinking.* New Haven: College and University Press, 1961.

Weiner, Jack B. *Drinking.* New York: W. W. Norton and Co., 1976.

The Whole College Catalog About Drinking. Washington, D.C.: U.S. Department of Health, Education and Welfare, 1976, 76–361.

Wilkenson, Rupert. *The Prevention of Drinking Problems: Alcohol Control and Cultural Influences.* New York: Oxford University Press, 1971.
Wilsnack, S. C. "The Effect of Social Drinking on Women's Fantasy." *Journal of Personality* 42 (1974): 43–61.
———. "The Impact of Sex Roles on Women's Alcohol Use and Abuse." Edited by M. Greenblatt and M. A. Schuckit. *Alcoholism Problems in Women and Children.* New York: Grune and Stratton, 1976.
———. "Sex Role Identity in Female Alcoholism." *Journal of Abnormal Psychology* 82 (1973): 253–61.
———, et al. "Drinking and Drinking Problems Among Women in a U.S. National Survey." *Alcohol Health and Research World* 9, no. 2 (Winter 1984/85): 11.
Wilson, G. T., et al. "Effects of Alcohol on Sexual Arousal in Women." *Journal of Abnormal Psychology* 85 (1976): 489–97.
Wiseman, J. P. "Spouses of Alcoholics." *Drugs, Alcohol and Women.* Washington, D.C.: National Institute on Drug Abuse—Program for Women's Concerns (October 24–26, 1975): 124–30.
Wolff, P. "Ethnic Differences in Alcohol Sensitivity." *Science* 175 (1972): 449–50.
Woman Alcohol Abuser: Subject Area Bibliography. Rockville, Md.: National Clearinghouse for Alcohol Information, 1974.
"Women: National Survey Data." *Alcohol Health and Research World.* Washington, D.C.: National Institute on Alcohol Abuse and Alcoholism, 9, no. 2 (Winter 1984/85).
Women: On Women in Recovery. St. Paul: Association of Half-Way House Alcoholism Programs in North America.
Wood, H. P., et al. "Psychological Factors in Alcoholic Women." *American Journal of Psychiatry* 123 (September 3, 1966): 341–45.
Yano, K., et al. "Coffee, Alcohol and Risk of Coronary Heart Disease Among Japanese Men Living in Hawaii." *New England Journal of Medicine* 297 (August 25, 1977): 405–09.
Young, James Harvey. *The Toadstool Millionaires.* Princeton: Princeton University Press, 1961.
Younger, William. *Gods, Men and Wine.* London: The Wine and Food Society, 1966.
Zucker, R. "Parental Influences Upon Drinking Patterns of Their Children." *Alcoholism Problems in Women and Children.* Edited by M. Greenblatt and M. A. Schuckit. New York: Grune and Stratton, 1976.

Index